Kinks and Fetishes Handbook

An A-Z Guide to Sexual Kinks, Fantasies and Fetishes, 50+ Freaky & Weird Sexual Fetishes, Kinks, and Terms You Should Absolutely Know plus Practical Tips on How to Go about Your Sexual Fantasies

Cheryl Bach

Kinks and Fetishes Handbook

Publisher: IntimateInk Press

Email: intimateinkpress@gmail.com

This book is a work of nonfiction intended for informational purposes only. The content of this book is based on the author's research, knowledge, and experience, and it is provided with the understanding that the author and publisher are not engaged in rendering legal, medical, or professional advice. The information in this book is not a substitute for professional guidance or assistance. Readers should consult with relevant professionals for advice and assistance regarding their specific situations. The author and publisher disclaim any liability for any loss or risk, personal or otherwise, which is incurred as a consequence, directly or indirectly, of the use and application of any of the contents of this book.

Cover design by IntimateInk Press

Interior layout and design by IntimateInk Press

Printed in USA

Fonts: Google fonts

Image: Freepik.com. This cover has been designed using assets from Freepik.com

For permission to use copyrighted material from this book, please contact the copyright holder listed above.

First Edition: 2024

Distributed by Amazon.com, Inc.

Table of Contents

Cheryl Bach

Table of Contents

Chapter 1

Introduction

The Kinks and Fetishes Handbook is a comprehensive guide to the world of sexual kinks, fetishes and fantasies. This book offers an A-Z list of sexual kinks, 50+ freaky and weird sexual fetishes, and an array of terms that individuals should know if they are interested in exploring this side of their sexuality. The book also provides practical tips on how to go about fulfilling one's sexual fantasies.

Sexual kinks and fetishes are an integral part of human sexuality. They represent unique interests and erotic desires that many people hold but may not be willing to discuss openly. Kinks and fetishes encompass a wide range of sexual preferences, ranging from mild to extreme. The beauty of kinks and fetishes is that they are so diverse, catering to every sexual preference imaginable.

Brief History of Kinks and Fetishes

The history of kinks and fetishes dates back centuries, with many ancient civilizations even practicing forms of BDSM and other kinks in sexual rituals and traditions. However, kinks and fetishes have been taboo topics for a long time, and many people feel hesitant to disclose their own kinks and fetishes, leading them to explore them in private.

In recent times, people have become more open to exploring their sexuality and accepting their kinks and fetishes as a natural part of themselves. The rise of the internet and social media has also made it easier for individuals to connect with others who share similar interests and desires.

Importance of Exploring and Accepting Individual Sexuality

The importance of exploring and accepting individual sexuality cannot be overstated. Understanding and accepting one's self is a crucial aspect of personal growth and development. By exploring their kinks and fetishes, individuals can enhance their sexual experiences, improve communication with their partners, and ultimately lead to a more fulfilling sex life. Accepting one's sexuality also removes the shame and judgment that has often surrounded kinks and fetishes in the past.

It is essential to remember that every individual has unique sexual desires, and it is entirely normal to have a kink or fetish. What counts is consensual exploration and communication with partners for a healthy and safe sex life.

This book aims to help individuals explore their kinks and fetishes in a safe, affirmative, and fun environment.

Whatever an individual's sexual preference, they can expect to gain valuable insights from this book regarding how to enhance their sex lives and reach further emotional and physical satisfaction.

So, buckle up and read through this book as we take you on an all-inclusive tour of kinks, fetishes, and fantasies!

Chapter 2

The Kinks Bible

In this chapter, we delve into the essential aspects of kinks and fetishes, providing definitions, a list of the most common kinks and fetishes, and the benefits of embracing them.

Definition of a Kink and Fetish

A kink refers to any unconventional sexual practice, interest, or activity that deviates from the commonly accepted societal norms. A fetish, on the other hand, involves experiencing sexual attraction or arousal from a non-sexual object or part of the body.

List of the Most Common Kinks and Fetishes

- **BDSM** – bondage, discipline, dominance, submission, sadomasochism

- **Exhibitionism** – sexual arousal from exposing oneself in public.

- **Voyeurism** – deriving pleasure from watching others engage in sexual activities.

- **Fetishism** – arousal from a particular object or body part, such as feet or leather.

- **Role-playing** – engaging in sexual playacting in different scenarios, such as doctor/nurse, teacher/student, etc.

- **Swinging** – engaging in consensual non-monogamous sexual activities with other couples or individuals.

- **Cuckolding** – deriving pleasure from watching one's partner have sex with someone else.

- **Bondage** – restraining someone during a sexual encounter for erotic purposes.

- **Impact play** – the use of instruments such as whips or paddles to create sensations of pain or pleasure.

- **Sensory deprivation** – intentionally reducing or removing an individual's sensory input, such as through blindfolds or earplugs, during a sexual activity.

How Kinks and Fetishes Differ from One Another

Kinks and fetishes vary greatly. While some practices may fall under both categories, there is a fundamental difference between kinks and fetishes. A kink refers to any activity that enhances sexual pleasure by deviating from the norm. In contrast, a fetish involves the need for specific objects or practices to achieve sexual arousal.

Benefits of Embracing Kinks and Fetishes

Embracing one's kinks and fetishes has several benefits. First and foremost, it fosters a healthier expression of one's sexual desires. Choosing to explore one's sexuality without judgment or fear helps in developing a healthy relationship with one's sexuality, leading to self-awareness, confidence, and self-acceptance.

It also enhances intimacy in relationships. When an individual chooses to reveal their kinks and fetishes to their partner, they allow them to fully understand their sexual experience and engage in activities that cater to their unique desires. Disclosure of fantasies and fetishes can also foster emotional intimacy in a relationship since it requires vulnerability in communication, which often increases trust and connection.

Exploring kinks and fetishes also provides an opportunity to expand and enrich one's sexual experience. Trying out different activities and engaging with partners who share and respect their desires can lead to heightened pleasure and satisfaction. It encourages experimentation, which may help individuals learn more about themselves sexually, develop new skills, and discover new preferences.

Embracing kinks and fetishes can also improve overall sexual health. Practicing safe and consensual sex promotes physical safety and can protect against unwanted sexual infections and pregnancy. Furthermore, exploring and accepting one's sexuality has been linked to improved mental health outcomes such as reduced stress and anxiety levels, increased confidence, and even better sleep.

Overall, embracing kinks and fetishes leads to the adoption of a healthy and responsible sexual lifestyle, which ultimately contributes to one's overall wellbeing.

In conclusion, kinks and fetishes can be viewed as alternative sexual practices or preferences that form an essential part of an individual's sexuality. While they may differ from the accepted societal norms, kinks and fetishes can offer exciting, pleasurable experiences that allow individuals to explore and express their unique sexual desires in consensual, safe ways. Through this chapter, we hope to have given you a comprehensive understanding of kinks and fetishes, highlighting their range, benefits, and how to safely and consensually explore them. The next chapter will focus on exploring various kinks and fetishes in detail, providing practical tips on how to approach and incorporate them into your sexual experiences.

Chapter 3

Different Kinks and Fetishes

Acrophilia

Acrophilia is a sexual kink or fetish that involves feeling intense arousal when in high places. This can manifest in a multitude of ways, including climbing tall buildings or structures, bungee jumping, skydiving, and other activities that offer a risk of falling or provide a sense of being high up. People with acrophilia often find the sensation of being exposed to great heights to be both thrilling and sexually stimulating.

While the exact origins of acrophilia are unknown, theorists suggest that it has to do with the body's response to adrenaline and heightened stimulation. Adrenaline is known to be a powerful aphrodisiac that can trigger feelings of arousal and excitement in the brain. When a person with acrophilia is exposed to a high or dangerous situation, their body responds by releasing adrenaline, which enhances and amplifies their sexual arousal. This can result in a heightened state of pleasure during sexual activities.

People with acrophilia often engage in activities such as rock climbing, hiking, urban exploration, and other high-risk activities that provide an elevated experience. Some may also incorporate acrophilic themes into their sexual activities, such as having sex on top of a tall building or engaging in sexual activities while suspended in the air.

It is important to note that while acrophilia can be exciting and pleasurable, it can also be dangerous if not practiced safely. Those with acrophilia should take proper safety precautions when engaging in high-risk activities to avoid injury or harm.

Acrophilia is often compared to another kink called "sploshing," which involves sexual arousal from messy substances like mud, cake icing, or food. Both acrophilia and sploshing involve seeking out particular sensations that result in arousal, and both fetishes are often perceived as being risky or dangerous.

Another comparable kink is "edgeplay," which involves engaging in sexual activities that push both partners to their physical or emotional limits. Like acrophilia, edgeplay can be dangerous if not practiced safely, and it often involves risk-taking behaviors that result in intense physical or emotional arousal for both partners.

Overall, acrophilia is an exciting and unique kink that offers a thrill-seeking, adventurous experience for those who pursue it. By taking proper safety precautions, those with acrophilia can safely explore their kink while enjoying the intense feelings of pleasure that come with it.

Algolagnia (arousal from pain)

Algolagnia is a sexual fetish or kink in which a person experiences sexual arousal from pain. The experience of pain can vary from person to person, with some individuals seeking out mild forms of pain such as light spanking or nipple clamps, while others may enjoy more intense forms of pain such as flogging or wax play.

While the exact origin of algolagnia is unknown, it is thought to be related to the release of endorphins in the brain. Endorphins are the body's natural painkillers, and they are released in response to pain. The release of endorphins can produce a feeling of pleasure and euphoria, which can lead to sexual arousal.

People who practice algolagnia may use a variety of tools and techniques to induce pain, such as whips, canes, or even their own hands. Some may incorporate elements of bondage or domination into their play to further enhance the power dynamic and sensation of pain. It is important to note that while pain can be a part of sexual play, it should always be consensual and negotiated beforehand to ensure both parties are comfortable with the level of pain involved.

Algolagnia is often compared to other BDSM-related kinks or fetishes, such as sadomasochism (S&M) or dominance and submission (D/s). Like algolagnia, these kinks involve elements of power exchange and can involve varying levels of pain as part of sexual play.

Another similar fetish is formicophilia, which involves sexual arousal from insects or other small creatures crawling over the body. While this fetishndoes not involve pain, it can involve a similar release of endorphins and a power dynamic, as the person being crawled on may feel powerless and at the mercy of the insects.

Overall, algolagnia is a kink that is often misunderstood and stigmatized due to its association with pain. However, with proper communication and consent between partners, it can be a fulfilling and enjoyable experience for those who practice it. It is important for those interested in this kink to do their research and establish boundaries and safe words beforehand to ensure a positive and consensual experience.

Bondage and Discipline (B&D)

Bondage and discipline, or B&D, is a kink within the BDSM community that focuses on restraining a partner and disciplining them through the use of physical or psychological stimulation. The practice of B&D can involve consensual power exchange, pain, and humiliation to varying degrees.

The practice of bondage often involves one partner being restrained using ropes, chains, cuffs, or other restraints. Once restrained, the dominant partner may proceed to discipline the submissive partner in a variety of ways, such as spanking, flogging, tickling, or sexual stimulation. This dynamic can be incredibly erotic for both partners as it requires trust, communication, and vulnerability.

The practice of bondage and discipline has its origins in a variety of cultures and traditions throughout history. It is often associated with BDSM, which gained mainstream attention in the 20th century through the publication of erotic literature such as the works of Marquis de Sade and the popularization of fetish-based clothing such as leather and latex.

B&D can take many forms and may be tailored to each individual couple's preferences and limits. Some may engage in light bondage and spanking, while others may delve into more extreme forms of restriction and punishment. It is important to note that all bondage and discipline activities should be discussed prior to engaging in them, and clear boundaries and safe words should always be established to prevent any potential harm.

B&D is often compared to similar kinks or fetishes, such as sadomasochism (S&M), domination and submission (D/s), and masochism. While these kinks may involve elements of restraint and punishment, B&D is focused primarily on restraining and disciplining the submissive partner.

S&M, on the other hand, involves both partners engaging in sadistic and masochistic activities, with each partner taking turns receiving and giving pleasure and pain. D/s involves a power exchange dynamic, with one partner taking on a dominant role and the other taking on a submissive role, but may or may not involve B&D activities. Masochism, meanwhile, involves sexual pleasure derived from receiving pain or humiliation.

B&D may also be compared to the kinks of shibari or kinbaku, which involve the art of Japanese rope bondage. While these practices may share some similarities, shibari and kinbaku are focused primarily on the skill and aesthetics of rope bondage rather than the discipline and power exchange dynamic found in B&D.

Corset Fetishism

Corset fetishism is a kink that involves sexual arousal from corsets or tight-laced garments. It may involve the wearing of corsets, the fascination with the effect it has on the body, or both.

Corsets are tight-fitting garments worn around the midsection, designed to shape and mold the body to an hourglass figure. Those with a corset fetish may enjoy wearing corsets themselves, seeing others wear them, or simply admiring the aesthetic of a tightly laced corset. The feeling of constriction may contribute to the BDSM dynamic, with the corset acting as a form of bondage.

Cheryl Bach

Corsets have been worn for centuries, primarily by women. Initially designed to provide support and create a fashionable silhouette, corsets became increasingly tighter and more restrictive in the 19th century, leading to their association with eroticism. In the Victorian era, tight-laced corsets were seen as a sign of high social status and femininity.

Corset fetishism can take many forms. Some may enjoy the feeling of wearing a corset themselves, while others may be turned on by seeing a partner wear a corset. The fetish may also involve the process of lacing up the corset, which may be seen as an intimate and erotic act. For some, corset fetishism may also be associated with domination and submission, as the tight-fitting garment may symbolize bondage and control.

Corset fetishism can be compared to other clothing-related fetishes, such as latex or leather fetishism. Like corset fetishism, these kinks involve an attraction to the physical articles of clothing and the way it shapes the body. However, corset fetishism is unique in that it is specifically focused on the corset garment, and the way it tightens and molds the waist and torso.

One other fetish that may be compared to corset fetishism is waist training, where individuals wear tightly laced corsets for extended periods of time with the goal of achieving a smaller waist size. While waist training may involve a similar physical sensation to corset fetishism, it is typically not associated with sexual arousal or BDSM dynamics.

Overall, corset fetishism is a unique fetish within the BDSM and kink communities, and can be enjoyed by those who are turned on by the aesthetic or physical sensations associated with corsets.

Coprophilia

Coprophilia, also known as scat fetishism, is a kink that involves sexual arousal from feces. This fetish may include playing with, smelling, or tasting fecal matter.

In the world of kinks and fetishes, coprophilia is one of the more taboo and stigmatized sexual preferences. Those with this fetish may enjoy the sensation of being humiliated or degraded through the act of defecation, or may simply find the smell or taste of feces arousing.

Some may engage in coprophilia as part of BDSM dynamics, with feces used as a form of degradation and domination. This can include acts such as toilet slavery, where a submissive partner is required to act as a toilet for a dominant partner.

The origins of coprophilia are not well understood, but it is known that humans have been fascinated with feces and bodily waste for thousands of years. There is evidence of various ancient cultures practicing coprophagia, or the eating of feces, as part of religious or spiritual rituals. It is unclear whether these practices were seen as taboo or fetishistic at the time.

In modern times, many with a coprophilia fetish engage in activities such as smearing feces on their bodies or engaging in scat play with a partner. This can include defecation on a partner's body, in their mouth, or directly onto the genitals or sexual organs.

Coprophilia is often compared to urophilia or erotic urine play, due to the association with bodily waste. However, while urophilia involves urine, which is generally viewed as less taboo and more socially acceptable, coprophilia is considered more extreme and illicit. Some may also compare coprophilia to other forms of BDSM-related degradation play, such as humiliation or objectification.

It is important to note that engaging in coprophilia can be dangerous if proper precautions are not taken. Fecal matter can contain harmful bacteria and parasites, and ingesting it can lead to serious illness or infection. Those engaging in scat play should take safety measures such as using gloves and thoroughly cleaning the area afterward.

In conclusion, coprophilia is a taboo and controversial fetish within the BDSM and kink communities. While it may be arousing for some individuals, it is important to engage in this activity safely and with the understanding and informed consent of all parties involved. It is also essential to recognize that this fetish is not for everyone and should not be forced upon anyone.

Crush Fetishism

Crush fetishism, also known as trampling, is a sexual fetish in which individuals experience sexual arousal and pleasure from watching or participating in the crushing and destruction of various objects, animals, or even people. The objects that are most commonly crushed include insects, fruit, food, and sometimes even toys.

There has not been much documentation on the origin of this fetishism, but it is said to have originated in Japan as part of the "hard crush" subculture in the 1990s. The term "hard crush" refers to the practice of crushing small animals, such as mice, rabbits, and small birds, for sexual gratification. While this practice is illegal and viewed as animal cruelty, some people still engage in it.

Crush fetishism has different practices that depend on the preferences of the individual, such as the type of object or animal being crushed, the material used to crush it, and the level of intensity involved. Some people prefer to watch others crush objects or animals, while others enjoy doing the crushing themselves.

There are also similarities between crush fetishism and other fetishes like foot fetishism and BDSM practices, as all involve physical domination and submission. However, it is important to note that consent plays a crucial role in BDSM activities, whereas crush fetishism lacks that element.

It is worth highlighting that while some individuals may find crush fetishism arousing, it is important to remember that engaging in anything non-consensual, illegal, or harmful to oneself, others or animals is not acceptable. It is important to seek out healthy avenues for exploring one's sexuality and fetishes that are safe and consensual for all parties involved.

Overall, crush fetishism or trampling may not be well-known or widely accepted, but it is a reality and a valid expression of one's sexuality for some individuals. It is important to practice empathy and understanding towards those with crush fetishism as long as it is practiced consensually and without harming animals, people, or oneself.

For those interested in exploring this kink, it is recommended to only use safe and non-harmful methods for crushing, such as using inanimate objects like food or toys, and always getting clear consent from all parties involved. Communicating boundaries and safe words should also be established to ensure a safe and pleasurable experience for all involved.

Exploring one's sexuality and fetishes can be a fun and rewarding experience, but it is vital to prioritize safety and respect for all involved.

Cuckold Fetishism

Cuckold fetishism is a type of sexual fetish where an individual feels sexually aroused at the thought of their partner having sex with someone else. The cuckold is typically a heterosexual male who takes pleasure in watching or being told about his female partner having sexual relations with another man.

The origin of cuckold fetishism can be traced back to the middle ages, where it was used as a form of punishment for men who were deemed inadequate in their ability to satisfy their wives sexually. The term "cuckold" originated from the Old French word "cucuault," meaning "cuckoo bird," which lays its eggs in another bird's nest.

In modern times, cuckold fetishism has evolved into a form of consensual non-monogamy. It is not uncommon for couples to engage in cuckolding as a way to spice up their sex lives and explore their fantasies in a safe and consensual manner. It is important to note that cuckolding should only be practiced with the consent of all parties involved.

There are many different practices associated with cuckolding, including watching one's partner have sex, participating in a threesome, or simply hearing about one's partner's sexual encounters with others. The cuckold is often submissive in this dynamic and may also enjoy humiliation, degradation, or other forms of BDSM play.

One similar fetish to cuckoldry is hotwifing, which involves a couple where the woman is the one who engages in sexual relations with others outside of the relationship. The main difference between the two is that hotwifing tends to be a more equal sharing of power and control within the relationship, whereas cuckoldry emphasizes one partner's submission to the other.

Another related fetish is voyeurism, which involves gaining sexual pleasure from watching others engage in sexual activity. However, the difference between voyeurism and cuckolding is that in voyeurism, the individual gains sexual pleasure from watching strangers, while in cuckolding, the arousal comes from watching one's own partner have sex with someone else.

It is important to remember that all sexual fetishes and kinks are valid expressions of sexuality, and as long as they are practiced safely and consensually, there is nothing wrong with exploring them. Communication and respect for boundaries between partners are essential to ensuring a positive and fulfilling experience for all parties involved.

For those interested in exploring cuckolding or any other fetish, it is important to communicate openly with partners, establish clear boundaries and safe words, and prioritize the physical and emotional safety of all parties involved.

Exhibitionism

Exhibitionism is a sexual fetish where an individual experiences arousal and pleasure from exposing their body or genitalia to others in public or private settings without being caught or punished. This can involve flashing, streaking, or engaging in sexual activity in public spaces such as parks or beaches. It can also include online exhibitionism, where individuals post naked or risque photos of themselves online for others to see.

The origins of this fetish are not well-known, but it is believed to have been around for centuries. Some psychologists suggest that it may be related to the desire for attention and validation, while others speculate that it stems from early sexual experiences in which the individual received positive reinforcement for exposing themselves.

Exhibitionism can manifest in a variety of ways, from simply wearing provocative clothing in public to intentional flashing and public sexual activity. It can also be practiced with the help of a partner, where the individual enjoys exposing their body or engaging in sexual acts in front of their consenting partner. The power dynamic in exhibitionism can vary widely, ranging from consensual non-consent scenarios where one partner forces the other to perform sexual acts in public, to more egalitarian and mutually agreed-upon arrangements.

One common misconception about exhibitionism is that it is always practiced by men. In fact, women can be exhibitionists as well and may take pleasure in exposing their body to others in public or sharing intimate photos or videos online.

One similar fetish to exhibitionism is voyeurism, which involves gaining sexual pleasure from watching others engage in sexual activity. The main difference between the two is that exhibitionism involves being the one who is watched or seen, while voyeurism involves being the one who is doing the watching.

Another related fetish is the desire for public humiliation and degradation, where the individual seeks to be humiliated or frowned upon by others in public spaces. This fetish may overlap with exhibitionism, as individuals who enjoy being exposed in public may also enjoy the humiliation and disapproval of others.

It is important to note that exhibitionism can be a risky fetish to engage in, as it can be illegal and carries the risk of arrest or punishment. It is essential to ensure that any exhibitionist acts are consensual, take place in private or designated settings, and do not involve non-consenting individuals.

For those interested in exploring exhibitionism or any other fetish, it is important to communicate openly with partners, establish clear boundaries and safe words, and prioritize the physical and emotional safety of all parties involved.

Foot Fetishism

Foot fetishism, also known as podophilia, is a sexual fetish where an individual experiences arousal and pleasure from feet. This can include touching, licking, kissing, smelling, or worshipping feet in various forms. Some individuals may also enjoy being trampled or stepped on by feet.

The origins of foot fetishism are not well-known, but it is believed to be a common fetish that has been around for centuries. Some psychologists suggest that it may be related to early sexual experiences involving feet, while others speculate that it stems from the association between feet and power or domination.

Foot fetishism can manifest in a variety of ways. Some individuals may enjoy receiving foot massages or pedicures, while others may prefer more submissive acts such as licking or kissing their partner's feet. The power dynamic in foot fetishism can vary widely, ranging from a more equal exchange of foot play to a dominant/submissive dynamic, where one partner controls the foot play activities.

One similar fetish to foot fetishism is shoe fetishism, where an individual experiences arousal and pleasure from shoes. This may involve touching, smelling, or wearing the shoes. Like foot fetishism, the origins of this fetish are not well-known, but it may also involve power and domination dynamics.

Another similar fetish is trampling, where an individual enjoys being stepped on or trampled by the feet of another person. This can be practiced alone or with a partner, and may involve bare feet or wearing shoes or boots.

It is important to note that foot fetishism, like any fetish or kink, is a valid expression of sexuality as long as it is practiced safely and consensually.

Cheryl Bach

Forniphilia

Forniphilia is a sexual fetish in which an individual experiences arousal and pleasure from being used as a piece of furniture for their partner or others. This can include being transformed into a piece of furniture such as a chair, table or stool, or being restrained in a way that restricts movement and creates the illusion of being a piece of furniture.

The origins of this fetish are not well-known. However, it is believed to be related to the desire for domination and submission. Forniphilia is often practiced within BDSM play, where the submissive partner is used as a human prop or piece of furniture for the dominant partner. The submissive partner may be physically restrained during the activity, wearing a mask or other piece of clothing to further create the illusion of an object.

Forniphilia can manifest in a variety of ways. The submissive partner may be required to remain still and silent for long periods of time, or they may be required to make specific shapes or positions to become a piece of furniture. The dominant partner may also use the submissive partner's body as a table, footstool, or even a chandelier.

One similar fetish to forniphilia is objectification, where a person is treated as an object instead of a person. This can include being used as a piece of furniture, but can also involve other forms of objectification such as being turned into a statue or figurine. Objectification may also involve dehumanizing language or actions.

Another similar fetish is mummification, where an individual is wrapped tightly in bandages or other materials to restrict movement and create a sense of helplessness. Like forniphilia, mummification may involve being used as a piece of furniture, but it can also involve other forms of BDSM play.

It is important to note that like any fetish or kink, forniphilia is a valid expression of sexuality as long as it is practiced safely and consensually. Communication with partners, negotiation of boundaries and safe words are crucial in BDSM activities including forniphilia. It is important to ensure that the submissive partner is not in physical discomfort or pain, and that they have a way to communicate with their dominant partner if needed.

Moreover, proper aftercare measures should be taken by both individuals regardless of their dominant or submissive roles. Both people must partake in post-play rituals like communication, cuddling and support to process the experience of the scene.

Furries

Furries are individuals who enjoy dressing up in anthropomorphic animal costumes or adopting animal personas in a sexual context. This fetish may involve role-playing as an animal character, wearing a costume or fur suit, or engaging in sexual activities with other individuals dressed as anthropomorphic animals.

The origins of this fetish are not well-known, but it has been around since the 1980s and is believed to have originated within the science-fiction and fantasy fan communities. The interest in animal role-play and anthropomorphic characters has also been fueled by various books, cartoons, and movies that feature such characters.

Furry culture incorporates a range of practices including art, literature, and music. A common practice in the furry community is the creation of "fursonas," which are personalized animal characters that represent oneself. Furries may also attend conventions and other events where they can meet others who share their interests, engage in role-playing games such as "LARP" or live action role-play and participate in other activities related to their fetish.

One key aspect of furry culture is the use of fur suits or costumes. These suits may be custom-made and can be quite complex, featuring detailed designs and even electronic elements. Wearing a fur suit allows individuals to fully embody their animal persona, which can be perceived as liberating and empowering.

Furries often identify themselves as members of a subculture that celebrates acceptance, creativity, and self-expression. They view their fetish as a means of exploring their identity and sexuality in a unique and fulfilling way. The fetish does not necessarily involve actual animals, and practitioners of this fetish and sexuality do not condone engaging in sexual activity with animals.

One similar fetish to furries is pet play, which involves acting like a pet animal or treating a partner like one. This can include wearing a collar, leash or other animal accessories, as well as acting out specific behaviors such as eating from a bowl or using a litter box.

Another similar fetish is plushophilia, which is a sexual attraction to stuffed animals. Similar to furries, individuals with this fetish may engage in role-playing and use stuffed animals as part of their sexual fantasies.

Furries, like any other fetish, should always be practiced consensually and safely. Communication, mutual respect and clearly defined boundaries are crucial in all BDSM related activities including furries. It is important to ensure that all individuals involved are comfortable, physically safe, and not coerced into behaviors that they do not want to engage in.

It is worth noting that this fetish continues to be misunderstood and stigmatized by society at large. Furries are often portrayed in a negative light in popular media, and in some cases have been falsely associated with zoophilia or bestiality, despite having nothing to do with these illegal activities. Due to this, many furries are hesitant to discuss their fetish or may feel ashamed about their interest.

However, with the rise of the internet and online communities, the furry subculture has become more visible and accepted. There are now a variety of websites and social media platforms where furries can connect with like-minded individuals, share artwork, and discuss their interests. The community also uses art festivals, conventions, and gatherings to showcase their talent and foster a sense of belonging.

In conclusion, furries are a niche fetish that has gained popularity due to its unique appeal.

Gaining fetish

Gaining fetish, also known as feederism, is the sexual fetish where one person gets turned on by eating or becoming larger, while another finds arousal in feeding, specifically feeding their partner. Individuals with a gaining fetish often fantasize about weight gain, either in themselves or their partners, and enjoy activities such as overeating, receiving massages, or watching food shows together.

The origins of this fetish are not well-known but it has gained some recognition since the 1960s as thinner body types made their debut in the Western world of media. Some people believe that it may have originated from the BDSM community, as practices such as domination and submission are often involved.

Gaining fetish involves a range of practices which may include weight-gain and overeating. People with a gaining fetish often prefer to have partners or individuals who are more receptive to the idea of gaining weight and becoming larger. This might involve overfeeding, feeding high-calorie or fatty foods, and other practices to encourage weight gain in their partner.

In some cases, gaining fetishists may find sexual gratification in eating large amounts of food themselves. This could be done through overeating, binge-eating or force-feeding. People with this fetish may also enjoy seeing themselves grow and find pleasure in fitting into smaller clothing sizes after having gained weight.

One major concern with gaining fetish is the potential health risks associated with intentional weight gain. It is important to practice the fetish in a safe and consensual manner while maintaining good physical and mental health, especially if the individual plans to gain significant amounts of weight.

One similar fetish to gaining fetish is inflation, which involves sexual fantasies about inflating the body to a larger size. This fetish can be achieved through a variety of means, including using air pumps, liquids or gases. Like feederism, inflation is a fetish that involves increasing the size of the body. However, the difference is that inflation focuses on achieving an exaggerated form of body expansion.

Another similar fetish is vore, or vorarephilia, which is the fetish of the desire to be eaten or consuming another person. While this may not seem related to gaining, some people may feel a sense of weight gain or fullness from consuming someone else or being consumed by someone else.

Despite its unusual nature, gaining fetish is a legitimate sexual preference for many people. It provides a way for individuals to indulge in their desires while experiencing pleasure from certain acts or practices. That said, it is important that people who engage in this fetish do so safely and with consent to avoid any potential harm.

Golden Showers

Golden showers, also known as urolagnia, is a sexual fetish where individuals derive pleasure or arousal from urinating on their partner or being urinated on by their partner. This fetish often involves the use of bodily fluids as a form of erotic stimulation and may be done in different settings such as indoors, outdoors, or in the shower.

The origins of golden showers are not clearly understood, but it has been practiced in various forms throughout history. It was first named and classified in the 19th century under the psychoanalytic study of human sexuality. However, urine and other bodily fluids have been used for sexual purposes throughout human history, and can be found throughout various mythologies and stories.

In terms of practices, golden showers are done in different ways depending on individual preferences. For some people, the act of urinating on their partner or being urinated on by their partner can be foreplay or the main sexual act. Some prefer to have the urine remain as a part of sexual play, while others prefer to clean up afterwards.

Golden showers can be performed in many different settings, such as during masturbation, during foreplay, or during sexual intercourse. For some, it may include drinking their partner's urine, while others may find pleasure in just watching their partner urinate. Safety is also a crucial aspect to consider as urine can carry bacteria that may lead to infections or other complications.

One similar fetish to golden showers is scat play, or coprophilia, which involves sexual arousal from feces. Scat play can involve activities such as defecation, smearing feces, or ingestion of feces.

Gooning

Gooning is a sexual fetish or kink that's been gaining popularity in recent years. It's the act of becoming completely lost in sexual pleasure, and it can be done both alone or in groups. The term "gooning" comes from the goofy expression that many people have on their faces when they are feeling intense pleasure.

Origin and Practices

The exact origin of gooning isn't known, but it's thought to have started in the online sex community. It's generally considered a modern phenomenon, with the rise of internet porn playing a significant role in popularizing the fetish. One of the defining characteristics of gooning is the use of visual stimulation, with pornography being the most common choice. Participants will often spend hours watching explicit videos, matching their breathing and movements with those on the screen until they're consumed by waves of sexual pleasure.

Gooners often describe the state of being lost in sexual pleasure as similar to a trance. They might stroke themselves for hours on end without ejaculating, or simply watch porn without touching themselves at all. Some gooners choose to use drugs or alcohol to intensify the experience, although this is discouraged by many communities due to the risks associated with substance abuse.

One common variation of gooning involves multiple people participating in a group setting. This can take many forms, from online forums and chat rooms to real-life meetups with like-minded individuals. Some group gooning sessions involve people stroking themselves in unison, while others simply watch each other and share fantasies.

Hedonism

Hedonism is a philosophy that celebrates pleasure, particularly sensual pleasure. It's the belief that life should be enjoyed and that pleasure can lead to happiness and fulfillment. In a sexual context, hedonism can manifest as a kink or fetish that prioritizes physical pleasure over emotional connection or attachment. Those who practice hedonism in a sexual context may prioritize exploring new sensations and experiences to maximize pleasure.

The concept of hedonism dates back to ancient Greece, where the philosopher Epicurus argued that pleasure is the ultimate goal of life. In modern times, hedonism is practiced as both a philosophy and a sexual kink. In the context of a sexual kink, hedonists may prioritize their own pleasure above all else and prioritize exploring new sensations and experiences. Some may engage in casual sex or seek out multiple partners in pursuit of pleasure, while others may focus on exploring their own bodies through solo play.

Practicing hedonism safely generally involves good communication skills, clear boundaries, and consent from all parties involved. Without these key elements, hedonistic practices can become harmful to those involved.

Hedonism shares similarities with other sexual kinks and fetishes that prioritize physical sensation over emotional connection. Kinks like sensory deprivation, wax play, and impact play can also be seen as hedonistic in nature, as they are focused on exploring the body and creating pleasurable sensations. That being said, hedonism differs from these other kinks in that it places a greater emphasis on the pursuit of pleasure above all else, rather than specific activities or stimulation methods.

In addition, hedonism shares similarities with other sexual practices that prioritize pleasure over emotional connection, such as casual sex or engaging in non-monogamous relationships. However, it's important to note that practicing hedonism does not necessarily mean engaging in these practices.

Overall, while hedonism may not be for everyone, it is a valid expression of sexuality and can lead to fulfilling and pleasurable experiences for those who practice it. As with any kink or fetish, communication, consent, and safety should always be prioritized to ensure that all parties involved are comfortable and enjoying themselves.

Impact Play

Impact play is a sexual kink that involves using physical impact, such as spanking, flogging, caning, or paddling, to create pleasure. It's often associated with BDSM and power exchange dynamics, as one partner takes on a more dominant or sadistic role while the other takes on a more submissive or masochistic role. The goal of impact play is to create a combination of pain and pleasure by stimulating the nerve endings in the skin and increasing blood flow to the area.

Impact play has been around for centuries and is prevalent in many different cultures and traditions. In Western culture, it has roots in BDSM and has been popularized in modern times by the BDSM community. While some engage in impact play as a standalone kink, it's often used in combination with other BDSM practices like bondage, dominance and submission, and more.

Participants in impact play often establish safe words and boundaries before engaging in the activity to ensure consent and avoid causing any unintentional harm. Many practitioners also make use of specialized instruments like whips, canes, and paddles to create specific sensations and establish power dynamics.

Impact play is similar to other BDSM kinks and fetishes that involve physical stimulation and power exchange dynamics. For example, cock and ball torture (CBT) and ball busting also involve physical impact to sensitive areas for a combination of pain and pleasure. Other types of sensation play, such as wax play and knife play, can also be seen as similar to impact play as they involve stimulating the senses through physical sensation.

Klismaphilia (enema fetish)

Klismaphilia, also known as an enema fetish, is a sexual kink that involves the use of enemas for pleasure and/or erotic stimulation. This kink can involve giving or receiving an enema, inserting fluids (usually water or soapy water) into the anus through a tube or nozzle in order to stimulate the rectum and colon. Klismaphiles may also enjoy the sensation of having their bowels emptied or may derive pleasure from the feeling of fullness that comes with retaining the enema.

Enemas have been used for hygiene, medical, and sexual purposes for centuries, with ancient Egyptians and Greeks using them to purify the body and cleanse the colon. In modern times, enemas are often used in the BDSM community as a form of kinky play or as part of medical fetishism. Enemas may also be used as a way to prepare for anal sex or other anal activities. Klismaphiles may enjoy a variety of different enema practices, from self-administered enemas to having a partner administer one for them. They may also enjoy variations in fluid temperature, volume, and pressure or may add other elements to their play such as restraints or anal toys.

Klismaphilia shares some similarities with other kinks and fetishes related to anal play and erotic stimulation, such as anal training and pegging. These kinks focus on the stimulation of the anus and rectum for sexual pleasure. However, klismaphilia differs from these kinks in that it specifically involves the use of enemas, which adds an additional element of physical sensation and stimulation.

In addition, klismaphilia has some similarities to medical fetishism, which involves a fascination with medical procedures and equipment. However, while medical fetishism may involve the use of enemas in a clinical setting, klismaphilia is focused on the sexual pleasure derived from enemas.

Cheryl Bach

Knife Play

Knife play is a kink or fetish that involves the use of knives or other sharp objects for erotic stimulation. This can range from simple teasing with a blade to more intense forms of play, including cutting the skin (also known as blood play). For those who enjoy knife play, the thrill comes from the danger and fear associated with having a sharp object so close to the body.

The origins of knife play are unclear, though it has been featured in literature and art throughout history. In modern times, it has gained popularity among BDSM enthusiasts as a form of edge play, which refers to activities that push boundaries and involve an increased level of risk. Those who engage in knife play may take a variety of precautions to ensure safety, such as using dull blades or practicing on areas of the body where major arteries and vital organs are not located. Consent and communication are crucial in any knife play scene, and it is important to establish clear boundaries and safe words beforehand.

Practitioners of knife play may enjoy a variety of different activities, from simply teasing or tracing the skin with a blade to more intense forms of play such as cutting or branding. The focus for many is on the psychological aspects of the kink, as well as the heightened sensations that come with the presence of danger.

Knife play shares some similarities with other forms of edge play, including fire play, breathe play, and needle play. All of these activities involve an increased level of risk and may push the boundaries of what some people consider "safe" BDSM practices. However, knife play is unique in its focus on the fear and danger associated with having a sharp object in close proximity to the body. It also differs from other forms of BDSM in that it involves an actual physical object, rather than just the body itself or other BDSM toys.

Knife play may also be compared to other forms of blood play, which involve drawing blood for erotic purposes. While knife play can include cutting the skin and drawing blood, it is not always necessary and many knife play scenes do not involve any bleeding at all.

Overall, knife play is a form of BDSM that is not for everyone but can be incredibly exhilarating and satisfying for those who practice it. As with any kink or fetish, communication, consent, and safety are essential. Educating oneself on safe knife play practices and seeking out experienced partners can help ensure a safe and enjoyable experience.

Latex and Rubber Fetishism

Latex and rubber fetishism is a kink or fetish that involves the wearing or appreciation of tight-fitting clothing made from rubber or latex. This can include full-body catsuits, rubber corsets, latex stockings, and any other kind of clothing made from these materials. Those who enjoy this fetish are often drawn to the sensual feeling of the rubber or latex against their skin, as well as the aesthetic appeal of the shiny, tight clothing.

While the origins of latex and rubber fetishism are unclear, it has gained popularity in recent decades among BDSM and kink enthusiasts. Practitioners may enjoy wearing tight-fitting latex or rubber clothing themselves, or watching others wear it in a sensual or BDSM context. Some may also enjoy incorporating other BDSM activities into their latex and rubber play, such as bondage or domination and submission.

Latex and rubber clothing require specialized care, as they can be easily damaged by heat, sunlight, and certain chemicals. Many people who own latex or rubber clothing invest in special conditioning products to keep their fetish wear looking and feeling its best.

Latex and rubber fetishism shares some similarities with other forms of clothing fetishism, in which individuals are aroused by specific types of clothing or materials. However, what sets latex and rubber fetishism apart is the physically restrictive nature of the clothing itself, which can add an extra layer of sensuality to the experience.

Another kink that may be compared to latex and rubber fetishism is spandex fetishism, in which individuals are aroused by tight-fitting clothing made from spandex.

Leather Fetishism

Leather fetishism, also known as leather culture or leatherism, is a sexual fetish that involves an erotic attraction to leather clothing, accessories, and lifestyle. People who practice leather fetishism engage in sexual activities while wearing or being surrounded by leather garments such as jackets, corsets, pants, boots, gloves, and other accessories like whips, belts, and chains. The fetish is often associated with BDSM practices but can exist independently.

The origin of leather fetishism can be traced back to the gay male subculture in the mid-twentieth century. The early leather scene was a way for queer men to express their masculinity and create a sense of community. However, over time, leather has become a popular fetish among people of all genders and sexual orientations. Today, there are leather clubs and events all over the world where people gather to celebrate their love for leather fetishism, engage in discussions, workshops, and parties.

Practices within leather fetishism can include wearing leather clothing during sexual activities, engaging in BDSM practices including bondage, domination, and discipline, as well as incorporating leather accessories and devices such as whips, restraints, and masks. Some individuals may also engage in role-play scenarios, such as teacher/student or master/slave dynamics, while others may simply enjoy the sensation and smell of leather.

Leather fetishism is often associated with BDSM practices, but it can exist independently. However, there are other kinks and fetishes that share some similarities. For example, latex fetishism involves an erotic attraction to clothing made of latex, similar to leather fetishism's attraction to leather.

Both kinks involve the use of a specific material and commonly incorporate bondage and sensory deprivation into their practices. Additionally, there may be some overlap with fur fetishism, where individuals are attracted to the sensation and texture of fur on their skin. Ultimately, while there are similarities between these kinks and fetishes, each has its unique practices and attractions.

For those interested in exploring leather fetishism, communication, and consent play a vital role. It's important to have open and honest conversations with your partner(s) about your interests, boundaries, and desires. This can include discussing what type of leather clothing or accessories you find attractive, your comfort levels with BDSM practices, and any specific scenarios or role-playing you may want to explore together.

Lactation fetish

Lactation fetish, also known as lactophilia or milk fetishism, is a sexual fetish that involves an erotic attraction to breastfeeding and lactating individuals. People who engage in this fetish may be aroused by the sight of lactation, the taste of breast milk, or the act of inducing lactation.

The origins of lactation fetishism are unclear, but it has been referenced in ancient medical texts and artwork. In modern times, the fetish has become more prevalent with the rise of online communities dedicated to it. Practices within lactation fetishism can include breastfeeding as part of a sexual encounter, drinking breast milk, and using breast pumps to simulate lactation. There are also those who practice inducing lactation through hormone therapy or other methods to fulfill their fetish.

Lactation fetishism is a relatively unique fetish, but there are some similar kinks and fetishes that share some elements. For example, adult nursing relationships (ANR) involve breastfeeding between consenting adults as a form of intimacy and bonding. This may or may not involve sexual activity but typically involves lactation. Additionally, some individuals may have a breast fetish or partialism which involves an erotic attraction to breasts.

As with any fetish or kink, communication and consent are crucial when engaging in lactation fetish practices. If you are interested in exploring this fetish, it's important to have open and honest discussions with your partner(s) about your desires, boundaries, and comfort levels.

Macro fetishism

Macro fetishism is a specific subtype of macrophilia and giantess fetishism where the focus is on size difference or growth. In this kink or fetish, one partner takes on the role of a giant, often compared to a movie monster or Kaiju, while the other partner acts as the smaller, weaker victim. The size ratio can range from a few inches to towering heights up to hundreds of feet tall.

The origin of the macro fetishism is unclear. However, it has been present in popular culture for a long time, with movies like 'Attack of the 50 Foot Woman' and 'Honey I Shrunk the Kids' contributing to its prevalence. In role-playing scenarios, macro fetishism can take many forms depending on the exact interests of the individuals involved. For example, some might enjoy causing destruction or chaos on a miniature scale, while others may want to focus on the power dynamic between the two partners.

Practitioners of macro fetishism enjoy the feeling of being dominated or empowered by their fictional size differences. They might engage in different acts such as lifting and carrying, crushing, and trampling. Some enthusiasts prefer to use special effects such as green screening to simulate the effect of one person towering over the other.

It is worth noting that macro fetishism has some similarities with other kinks such as height difference, domination and submission, and size fetishism. While these kinks share some elements with macro fetishism, they each have their own unique flavors and can be practiced in different ways.

Height difference, for example, focuses on the height disparity between two individuals, but without necessarily involving growth or transformation. Domination and submission, on the other hand, may focus more on the power dynamics between two individuals, without necessarily involving size play. Size fetishism is more about the specific attraction to body size or shape than it is about the dynamic between two partners.

In conclusion, Macro fetishism is a fascinating and complex kink that allows partners to explore themes of power, dominance and submission, and size difference. While this kink might seem extreme to some, for those who practice it, it can provide a unique form of pleasure and an escape from reality. As with any kink, communication and consent are crucial, as it's important for both partners to feel comfortable and safe with the activities they engage in. Practicing macro fetishism requires communication, especially around boundaries and limits. Finally, practical tips on how to go about this kink or fetish include setting up safe words, creating rules of engagement, and understanding the effects of size difference-related experiences on the relationship.

Masochism

Masochism is a kink or fetish that involves deriving pleasure or sexual excitement from experiencing pain or humiliation. This desire for pain can be physical, emotional, or both. Masochists may enjoy being restrained, spanked, humiliated, or otherwise physically dominated by their partner.

The term masochism comes from the name of Leopold von Sacher-Masoch, a 19th-century Austrian author who wrote about this kind of behavior in his novels. However, the practice of masochism has been present in human sexuality for centuries. Like many other kinks and fetishes, the origin of masochism is still unclear, but some believe that it may be rooted in childhood experiences, emotional or psychological trauma, or even genetic predispositions.

Practices associated with masochism can vary greatly, depending on individual preferences and the extent to which they enjoy pain. This kink or fetish may involve activities such as spanking, bondage, humiliation, wax play, or needle play. Others may prefer to engage in role-playing scenarios where one partner takes on a dominant role, while the other embraces their submissive side.

While masochism might seem similar to sadism, both involve the enjoyment of receiving and inflicting pain, respectively, there are crucial differences between these two kinks. Masochists enjoy receiving pain, while sadists enjoy giving it.

Masochism is also often compared to submission and domination, as these kinks also involve power dynamics in a sexual context. However, submission and domination are not necessarily about physical pain or humiliation, but rather about the exchange of power and control between partners.

It's important for those who practice masochism to communicate clearly with their partners, and to trust one another. Establishing boundaries and limits before engaging in any kind of play is crucial, and should always be respected. Additionally, it's essential to have a "safe word" in place, which can be used to signal when activities have surpassed the intended limit.

Practicing masochism is not without its risks, and safety should always be a top priority. Any physical activity that involves pain, especially with instruments like needles or knives, should be done with extreme caution and after receiving proper training or education.

Finally, it's important to remember that masochism, like any other kink or fetish, is not indicative of an unhealthy psyche or damaged personality. It's simply a way that some people choose to express their sexuality and explore new aspects of themselves and their sexuality.

In conclusion, Masochism is a kink or fetish that involves deriving pleasure or sexual excitement from experiencing pain or humiliation. This kink or fetish has been present in human sexuality for centuries and can be sometimes rooted in childhood experiences, emotional or psychological trauma, or even genetic predispositions. Masochists may enjoy being restrained, spanked, humiliated, or otherwise physically dominated by their partner. Safety and communication are crucial when practicing masochism, as well as establishing boundaries and limits before engaging in any kind of play.

Medical Fetishism

Medical fetishism is a kink or fetish that involves the sexual use of medical instruments, procedures, and environments. People who practice this kink gain sexual pleasure and/or excitement from the sensations and experiences of being treated medically. This may include activities such as role-playing as medical professionals like doctors or nurses, wearing medical costumes, or even imitating medical procedures.

The origin of medical fetishism is unknown, but some believe it can be linked to the feeling of vulnerability and taboo that arises from being in a hospital setting. However, medical fetishism can also develop from a fascination with the human body and its functions. People who are drawn to this kink may seek out other people who share their interest in the medical field and engage in activities that mimic medical procedures, such as injection play and catheterization.

Despite being a somewhat taboo fetish, medical role-play can be enjoyed safely with clear communication and role-playing materials. It's essential to establish boundaries and limits beforehand and ensure that all parties involved are comfortable with their roles and responsibilities. Medical fetishists also often use sterile instruments and medical-grade equipment, which reduces the risk of spreading harmful bacteria and infections.

Medical fetishism is often compared to BDSM and bondage, as well as erotic enema play. However, BDSM focuses on pain and submission as sources of sexual pleasure, while medical fetishism focuses more on examination and care. Bondage in medical fetishism is less about restriction and more about physical examination and manipulation.

Erotic enema play involves the use of enemas for sexual pleasure, which could be seen as a part of medical fetishism because enemas are often used for medical reasons.

However, erotic enema play focuses more on the sensations of the enema itself rather than the overall medical experience.

In summary, medical fetishism is a kink or fetish that involves the use of medical instruments, procedures, and environments for sexual pleasure and excitement. It can develop from a fascination with the human body, a taboo curiosity associated with medical environments, or a combination of both. Clear communication and playing safe is crucial and following universal health-precautions like using sterile instruments and medical equipment reduces the risk of infections.

Mummification

Mummification is a kink or fetish that involves wrapping a person, usually nude, in materials like plastic wrap, duct tape, or bandages, depriving them of movement and sensation. People who practice this kink report feeling a sense of vulnerability and loss of control, which they find erotic and pleasurable. Mummification can also be combined with other kinks, like sensory deprivation or bondage.

The origins of mummification as a kink are unclear but it is believed that it emerged from the Ancient Egyptian practice of mummifying the dead. The practice of binding, wrapping or encasing living individuals in materials is thought to date back to ancient times for ceremonial or spiritual purposes.

In modern mummification practices, people use materials like plastic wrap or duct tape to create a "cocoon" around the body. Some practitioners may even use vacuum-sealed bags to encase the entire body and heighten the sense of confinement. The process can take up to several hours, and once complete, the person is unable to move or speak. Safety is paramount in mummification play. It's important to avoid wrapping the face and to make sure that the individual being mummified can still breathe freely. Using a safe word or signal is also vital to communicate in case of any discomfort or emergencies.

Mummification is often compared to other forms of bondage, such as rope bondage or shibari, as it involves a similar sense of restraint and loss of control. However, mummification is distinguished by the use of tight materials that can create a complete, cocoon-like experience. Some people combine mummification with sensory deprivation, where the encased person is unable to see, hear, or speak. This intensifies the feeling of helplessness and submission.

Another kink that may be considered similar to mummification is encasement fetishism, where people are sexually aroused by being enclosed in materials like spandex, latex, or leather. However, encasement usually allows for more movement and flexibility than mummification, and often involves the wearing of a suit or garment rather than being wrapped or encased in a material.

Object Fetishism

Object fetishism is a kink or fetish that involves sexual attraction or arousal to certain objects. People who practice this fetish may have a strong sexual desire for a particular object like shoes, clothes, or toys, to the extent that it becomes a sexual fixation. This fetish can also involve a focus on specific textures, colors, or materials.

The origins of object fetishism are unclear, but it is believed to be a component of human sexuality experienced by a small percentage of individuals. This fetish can emerge based on early-life experiences or associations formed in childhood, or it can be a result of the individual's unique psychological makeup and sexual orientation.

In object fetishism practices, people may incorporate objects as part of their sexual activities, such as using certain objects during masturbation or incorporating them into sexual play with their partners. They may derive sexual pleasure from looking at or touching the object, as well as using or smelling it in sexual activity.

It's important to note that object fetishism does not involve any harm to oneself or others, and it is often a consensual and harmless activity. However, as with any kink or fetish, communication and mutual consent are essential for a safe and enjoyable experience.

Object fetishism can be compared to other fetishes like shoes or clothing fetishism, but the focus in object fetishism is on the object itself rather than the clothing or shoes as an accessory for the human body. However, some people may have a mix of both fetishes.

Another fetish that is similar to object fetishism is plushophilia, which involves sexual attraction or arousal to stuffed animals or plush toys. Like object fetishism, it is focused on a specific object and can involve using the object as part of sexual activity.

In summary, object fetishism is a kink or fetish that involves sexual attraction or arousal to specific objects such as shoes, clothes, or toys. This fetish can emerge based on early-life experiences, unique psychological makeup, or other factors, and practitioners incorporate objects into their sexual activities to derive pleasure. It is important to emphasize that this fetish is harmless as long as it is practiced consensually and safely.

Omorashi (bladder desperation)

Omorashi is a kink or fetish that involves sexual arousal from bladder desperation or the act of holding one's urine. People who practice this fetish may derive pleasure from the feeling of fullness and pressure in their bladder, as well as the release and relief of urinating after holding it in.

The origins of omorashi are unclear, but it is believed to have originated in Japan and is often associated with anime and manga culture. In practice, people may enjoy engaging in activities like drinking large amounts of fluids to increase their desperation, wearing clothing that restricts urination, or engaging in power play scenarios where one partner controls when the other can or cannot go to the bathroom.

Some people may also enjoy watching others engage in bladder desperation, whether in person or through videos or photos. It's important to note that consent and communication are essential in any sexual activity, including omorashi. Partners should agree on methods, boundaries, and safety precautions before engaging in this fetish.

Omorashi can be compared to other fetishes like urophilia (water sports) or scatophilia (fecal play), but it does not always involve actual bodily fluids like urine or feces. Instead, the focus is on the feeling of holding and releasing urine. However, some people may also incorporate elements of these other fetishes into their omorashi play.

In summary, omorashi is a kink or fetish that involves sexual arousal from bladder desperation or the act of holding one's urine. It may have originated in Japan and can involve activities like drinking large amounts of fluids, wearing restrictive clothing, or engaging in power play scenarios. Partners should always communicate and agree on boundaries and safety measures before practicing this fetish. Omorashi can be compared to other fetishes like urophilia and scatophilia but is focused on the feeling of holding and releasing urine rather than bodily fluids themselves. Like any kink or fetish, omorashi is a personal preference and consenting adults should feel free to explore it in a safe and consensual manner.

Olfactophilia (arousal from smells)

Olfactophilia is a kink or fetish that involves sexual arousal or attraction to smells. People with this fetish may derive pleasure from a wide range of scents, including body odors, perfumes, pheromones, or even specific objects like shoes or clothing. They may enjoy sniffing or licking body parts, inhaling partners' scents, or using scented products during sexual activities.

The exact origins of olfactophilia are unknown, but it is likely related to our evolutionary past as smell plays a key role in sexual attraction and mating behavior in many species. However, it is important to note that not everyone experiences or shares this fetish, and it can emerge based on individual preferences, experiences, or unique psychological makeup.

In practice, olfactophilia can involve a variety of practices like body odor worship, scent fetishism, or wearing specific fragrances during sexual activities. Some people may also enjoy engaging in role-playing scenarios like "sweaty gym" or "dirty panties" to enhance the sensory experience. It is important to note that all activities should be consensual and agreeable to both parties.

Olfactophilia can be compared to other fetishes like foot fetishism or hair fetishism, which also focus on specific body parts or attributes. However, the key difference is that olfactophilia centers on smells rather than physical attributes. It can also be compared to urophilia, fecal fetishism, or other fetishes that involve bodily fluids, as scents are also a means of transmitting and signaling sexual attraction and arousal. However, olfactophilia does not necessarily involve the exchange of bodily fluids and can focus on a wide range of smells.

It is important for people with olfactophilia to communicate their preferences and boundaries with their partners before engaging in sexual activities. While this fetish may not be considered "mainstream," it is still a valid and consensual way for individuals to experience sexual pleasure. When practiced in safe and respectful ways, olfactophilia can enhance sexual intimacy and satisfaction for all parties involved.

In summary, olfactophilia is a kink or fetish that involves sexual arousal or attraction to smells. It can involve a variety of practices like body odor worship, scent fetishism, and using specific fragrances during sexual activities. It may have originated from the evolutionary role that smells play in sexual attraction and mating behavior, but it can also emerge from individual preferences or unique psychological makeup. Communication and consent are essential when engaging in olfactophilia, as with any fetish or kink. While it may be compared to other fetishes like foot or hair fetishism and urophilia or fecal fetishism, the focus on smells sets it apart. Ultimately, olfactophilia is a valid and consensual way for individuals to experience sexual pleasure when practiced safely and respectfully with consenting partners.

Cheryl Bach

Orgasm control

Orgasm control, also known as orgasm denial or edging, is a kink or fetish that involves the manipulation and management of sexual release. People who practice orgasm control may enjoy the heightened sexual tension and anticipation that comes from delaying or denying orgasm, often using specific techniques and tools to prolong the experience.

The origins of orgasm control are unclear, but it has been practiced by individuals and couples for centuries. Some people may be drawn to this fetish because they enjoy the psychological aspect of control, while others may thrill in the physical sensations and heightened arousal of edging. Orgasm control can be practiced in a variety of ways, including through masturbation, manual stimulation, or the use of sex toys.

One common practice for orgasm control is "edging," where a person approaches the brink of an orgasm but stops or slows down stimulation before it happens, repeatedly building up and reducing sexual tension. Other techniques may involve using a specific countdown, verbal commands, or physical restraints to delay orgasm or heighten sexual sensations.

Orgasm control can be compared to other kinks or fetishes that involve aspects of control, such as bondage or dominance and submission (D/s) roleplay. However, the specific focus on orgasm and sexual release sets orgasms control apart from other practices. It also often emphasizes a collaborative dynamic between partners, as communication and negotiation are essential to ensure both parties are comfortable and enjoying the experience.

It's important to note that orgasm control can have both physical and emotional benefits. By delaying orgasm, people may experience more intense pleasure when they finally do reach climax. This can result in stronger, more satisfying orgasms. Additionally, some people may enjoy the psychological thrill of relinquishing control and submitting to their partner's desires.

However, it's also important to practice orgasm control safely and with clear communication between partners. Extended periods of stimulation without release can cause discomfort or pain, and should be avoided. Additionally, it is important to establish clear boundaries and safe words to ensure all parties are comfortable and enjoying the experience.

In summary, orgasm control is a kink or fetish that involves the manipulation and management of sexual release. It can be practiced in a variety of ways and emphasizes collaborative communication and negotiation between partners. While it may offer physical and emotional benefits, it is important to engage in safe practices and establish clear boundaries. People interested in exploring orgasm control can communicate their fantasies and desires with their partners and experiment with different techniques, such as edging or using sex toys. Ultimately, orgasm control can be a fun and exciting way for individuals to explore their sexual desires and experience heightened pleasure through delayed gratification.

Ponyplay

Ponyplay is a kink or fetish that involves roleplaying as a horse or other pony-like animal. It generally involves a dominant partner acting as the "handler" and a submissive partner acting as the "pony," with the submissive partner wearing gear such as a bit gag or harness to help simulate the experience. Ponyplay can be practiced in a variety of different ways, but typically involves training and conditioning the submissive partner to behave like a horse, including performing actions like neighing, walking on all fours, and pulling a cart or carriage.

The origins of Ponyplay as a fetish are unclear, though it has been suggested that it may have originated from the practice of animal roleplay, particularly with bondage enthusiasts. Ponyplay is often enjoyed for its emphasis on power dynamics and submission, as well as for the unique experience of acting out animalistic behaviors.

Practices for Ponyplay can vary widely, depending on the interests and preferences of the participants. Some individuals may engage in light ponyplay, incorporating only selected gear such as tails or ears, while others may engage in full-body coverings or elaborate costumes to simulate the appearance of a pony. Ponyplay can also include training sessions, where handlers train the ponies through various exercises and commands.

Ponyplay can be compared to other types of animal roleplay, such as puppy play or kitten play, but differs in the focus on equine behavior and anatomy. Additionally, Ponyplay often places a greater emphasis on the power dynamics and control between the handler and pony, as well as on the physical sensations and movements of the submissive partner.

It's essential to practice safe and consensual Ponyplay, with both partners agreeing to boundaries, safe words, and other safety measures. Handlers should ensure that their ponies are physically comfortable and free from harm, while also providing proper training and conditioning to help them achieve the desired roleplay experience.

People interested in Ponyplay can find gear and equipment from specialist suppliers and online retailers, including bits, harnesses, tails, and hoof boots. They may also participate in Ponyplay events or contests, where they can meet like-minded individuals and showcase their skills, costumes, and accessories.

In summary, Ponyplay is a kink or fetish that involves roleplaying as a horse or pony-like animal, with a dominant partner acting as a handler and a submissive partner acting as a pony. It can involve various forms of training and conditioning, costume or gear, and power dynamics. While Ponyplay is not for everyone, those who enjoy it can find a unique experience that emphasizes submission and animalistic behaviors. As with any other kink or fetish, it is important to engage in safe and consensual practices, communicate openly with partners, and establish clear boundaries and safety measures.

Cheryl Bach

Power Exchange

Power Exchange is a kink or fetish that involves a consensual exchange of power between partners, where one partner takes control over the other. This exchange of power can range from subtle power-play dynamics to more explicit Dominant/submissive roleplay. Power Exchange typically involves trust, obedience, and a willingness to explore the power dynamics within a relationship, often with the aim of enhancing sexual pleasure and intimacy.

The origins of Power Exchange as a fetish are difficult to trace, but many scholars believe it has roots in BDSM culture and other related fetishes involving Dominant/submissive power dynamics. Power Exchange can be practiced in various ways, such as in a 24/7 committed relationship where one partner assumes a dominant role and the other a submissive one, or in a casual sexual encounter where partners take on specific roles during the encounter.

Practices for Power Exchange can include exploring the boundaries of submission and domination, engaging in discipline and punishment, and creating elaborate power exchange scenarios that satisfy the desires of both partners. For example, a Dominant partner may use physical restraint or verbal cues to control their submissive partner's movements or behavior, while the submissive partner may be rewarded for obedience or punished for disobedience.

Power Exchange can be compared to other BDSM kinks such as bondage or spanking, but differs in the focus on power dynamics and control within a relationship. Additionally, Power Exchange is more concerned with the psychological and emotional aspects of control and submission, rather than just the physical sensations.

It is important for partners engaged in Power Exchange to establish clear boundaries, safe words, and other safety measures, as well as to communicate openly about their desires and expectations. In many cases, Power Exchange can be a mutually beneficial kink that enhances intimacy and sexual pleasure for both partners, but it must be practiced safely and with clear consent.

People interested in Power Exchange can find resources and information from BDSM communities and online forums, as well as from specialized books and guides that explore the topic in greater depth. They may also participate in BDSM events or workshops, where they can learn more about Power Exchange and meet like-minded individuals who share their interests.

In conclusion, Power Exchange is a unique and complex kink that involves the consensual exchange of power between partners. It can range from subtle power-play dynamics to more explicit Dominant/submissive roleplay, and it often emphasizes trust, obedience, and psychological and emotional aspects of control. It is important for partners to communicate openly, establish clear boundaries and consent, and practice safe and responsible Power Exchange in order to enhance intimacy, pleasure, and connection within their relationship. While Power Exchange may not be for everyone, those who explore this kink can find a rewarding and fulfilling experience that enhances their sexual and emotional connection with their partner.

Pregnancy fetishism

Pregnancy Fetishism is a kink or fetish that involves sexual attraction to pregnant women or the idea of impregnation. This fetish can manifest in various ways, such as fantasizing about pregnancy, watching pregnant pornography, or engaging in roleplay scenarios involving pregnancy. Some individuals with this fetish may also engage in lactation-based fantasy or enjoy the physical signs of pregnancy, such as increased breast size or a swollen belly.

The origin of Pregnancy Fetishism is not easy to trace, but some scholars believe it is connected to the desire for sexual reproduction and the evolutionary drive to procreate. Others believe it may be tied to cultural or societal beliefs about fertility and motherhood. Practices for Pregnancy Fetishism include engaging in roleplay scenarios that involve a partner who is pregnant, or who wishes to become pregnant. This can involve wearing a prosthetic pregnancy belly, or using erotic language related to pregnancy and childbirth during sex.

Pregnancy Fetishism can be compared to other fetishes that involve specific physical characteristics or attributes, such as breast or foot fetishism. However, it is important for individuals with this fetish to approach their desires with sensitivity and respect for pregnant women, and to recognize the unique physical and emotional challenges that pregnant women face. It is also important to remember that non-consensual actions related to this fetish, such as uninvited touching or comments towards pregnant women, can be harmful and disrespectful to their autonomy and well-being.

Individuals with Pregnancy Fetishism may benefit from seeking out the company of others who share their fetish, such as through online forums or social media groups. This can provide a safe space to explore their desires, share fantasies, and connect with others who understand their feelings. It is also important for individuals with this fetish to communicate openly with their partners about their desires and boundaries, and to ensure that any roleplay scenarios involving pregnancy are conducted with clear consent and respect.

Overall, Pregnancy Fetishism is a kink or fetish that involves sexual attraction to pregnancy and the physical and emotional changes associated with it. As with any fetish, it is important to approach desires with sensitivity and respect, to communicate openly with partners, and to ensure that all actions are consensual and respectful.

Pyrophilia (fire fetish)

Pyrophilia, also known as fire fetish or pyromania, is a kink or fetish that involves sexual arousal from fire or other related elements. Individuals with this fetish may experience sexual pleasure through watching a fire burn, feeling the heat of a flame against their skin, or playing with fire during sex. This fetish can be risky, as it involves engaging with a potentially dangerous element, and should only be practiced with extreme caution and careful consideration.

The origin of Pyrophilia is not well understood, but it is thought to be linked to a desire for danger and excitement, as well as a fascination with natural elements. Practices for Pyrophilia can include lighting candles or fires during sex, using hot wax or heated objects as part of BDSM play, or engaging in fire or candle wax play.

Pyrophilia can be compared to other kinks or fetishes that involve exploring sensory experiences, such as BDSM or rope bondage. However, it is important to note that this fetish also involves a potentially dangerous element, and should only be practiced by individuals who are knowledgeable about fire safety and have taken proper precautions.

Individuals with Pyrophilia may benefit from seeking out communities or online forums dedicated to this fetish in order to connect with others who share their desires and find safe ways to explore them. It is important for individuals with this fetish to always prioritize safety above all else, communicate openly with partners about boundaries and desires, and to never engage in potentially risky behavior while under the influence of drugs or alcohol.

It is also important to note that, while Pyrophilia can be a consensual and enjoyable fetish for some individuals, it can also be dangerous and non-consensual behavior should never be tolerated. It is important to ensure that all activities related to this fetish are conducted with clear and informed consent from all parties involved.

Overall, Pyrophilia is a kink or fetish that involves sexual attraction to fire or other related elements. While it can provide a unique and exciting experience for some individuals, it should only be practiced with extreme caution and careful consideration, and always with safety as the top priority. As with any fetish or kink, it is important to communicate openly with partners, respect boundaries, and ensure that all activities are conducted with clear and informed consent.

Cheryl Bach

Quicksand fetish

Quicksand fetish, also known as mire or mud fetish, is a kink or fetish that involves sexual arousal from the idea of sinking into quicksand or mud. Individuals with this fetish may be aroused by imagining or watching others sink into these substances, or may enjoy engaging in this kind of play during BDSM scenes.

The origin of this fetish is unknown, but it is thought to be linked to a desire for power dynamics or submission, as well as the tactile sensation of being immersed in soft, sticky substances. Practices for this fetish can include roleplaying scenarios where one partner is "stuck" in quicksand or mud, or simply incorporating these substances into traditional BDSM scenes.

Quicksand fetish can be compared to other kinks or fetishes that involve tactile sensations or power dynamics, such as sensory deprivation play or pet play. However, it is important to note that this fetish involves an element of physical danger, and should only be practiced with extreme caution and careful consideration.

Individuals with this fetish may benefit from seeking out communities or online forums dedicated to this fetish in order to connect with others who share their desires and find safe ways to explore them. It is important for individuals with this fetish to prioritize safety by researching the safest ways to engage in quicksand or mud play, and creating clear boundaries and safe words with their partners.

It is also important to note that, while Quicksand fetish can be a consensual and enjoyable fetish for some individuals, it can also be dangerous, and care should be taken to ensure that all activities related to this fetish are conducted with clear and informed consent from all parties involved.

Rimming

Rimming, also known as analingus, is a sexual activity that involves oral stimulation of the anus. This can include using the tongue, lips, or teeth to stimulate the external and internal parts of the anus and surrounding area. Individuals with this fetish may experience pleasure from performing or receiving rimming, or may find it to be a turn-on as part of a wider kink or fetish.

The origin of rimming is unclear, but it has been depicted in various forms of art and literature throughout history. Practices for this fetish can include incorporating rimming into foreplay or sex, or using it as part of BDSM play. It is important to note that rimming can also involve the transmission of STIs and other health risks, and should be practiced with care and thorough communication between partners.

Rimming can be compared to other kinks or fetishes that involve anal play, such as pegging or prostate stimulation. However, rimming specifically involves oral stimulation of the anus and surrounding area and may be more focused on the sensory experience and vulnerability associated with that act.

Individuals with this fetish may benefit from seeking out communities or online forums dedicated to rimming in order to connect with others who share their desires and find safe ways to explore them. It is important for individuals engaging in rimming to prioritize hygiene and communication, setting clear boundaries and discussing any potential health risks with their partners beforehand.

Overall, rimming is a kink or fetish that may involve sexual arousal from oral stimulation of the anus and surrounding area. While it can provide a unique and exciting experience for some individuals, it should only be practiced with extreme caution and careful consideration, and always with safety as the top priority.

Role play

Role play, also known as erotic role play or sexual role play, is a kink or fetish that involves acting out specific scenarios, often with costumes, props, and dialogue, in order to create a sexual fantasy. These scenarios can range from innocent to taboo, and may involve power dynamics, dominance and submission, or other forms of fantasy.

The origin of role play is unclear, but it has been depicted in various forms of media throughout history, and has likely existed in some form for centuries. Practices for this fetish may involve visual or intellectual stimulus, such as wearing costumes or engaging in intellectual banter, as well as physical stimulus, such as bondage or sensory deprivation.

Role play can be compared to other kinks or fetishes that involve creating immersive sexual experiences, such as BDSM or sensory play. However, the focus of role play specifically is on creating a dynamic or narrative that allows individuals to live out sexual fantasies in a safe and consensual way.

Individuals with this fetish may benefit from seeking out communities or online forums dedicated to role play in order to connect with others who share their interests and find safe ways to explore them. It is important for individuals engaging in role play scenarios to communicate clearly with their partners about boundaries and desires, and to establish safe words or signals to indicate when a scenario should be stopped.

Overall, role play is a kink or fetish that can offer a fun and exciting way to explore sexual fantasies and experiment with power dynamics and sensory experiences. While it is important to always prioritize safety and clear communication, individuals engaging in role play may find that it opens up new pathways for sexual exploration and enjoyment.

Sadism

Sadism is a kink that involves deriving pleasure through inflicting pain on others. It involves the desire to control or dominate others, often involving bondage, humiliation, impact play, and other forms of physical or emotional abuse.

The origins of sadism can be traced back to the Marquis de Sade, a French aristocrat and writer who lived from 1740 to 1814. He authored many books that explored themes of sadomasochism, including "120 Days of Sodom" and

"Justine". Sadism has evolved through the years and is now one of the most common kinks in the BDSM community.

Practitioners of sadism enjoy manipulating and controlling their partners. They often have a strong desire to dominate and make their partner submit to their will. The dynamic of the dominant/submissive relationship is key to sadism, and trust and communication are crucial for safe and consensual play.

Similar kinks to sadism include masochism and bondage. Masochism involves deriving pleasure from being the recipient of pain and humiliation, while bondage involves being restrained or tied up for sexual pleasure. Both of these kinks can often be combined with sadism to create a power dynamic within the relationship.

Whether or not you're into sadism, it's important to remember that everyone has their own unique sexual desires and fantasies. It's important to be non-judgmental and accepting of others' kinks and identities, as long as it is safe, legal, and consensual. By being open-minded, respectful, and communicative, we can create a more inclusive and fulfilling sexual community for everyone.

In summary, sadism is a kink that involves the desire to dominate and control one's partner through inflicting pain and/or humiliation. It originated from the works of Marquis de Sade and has evolved throughout the years. It can be practiced safely and consensually by establishing clear communication, boundaries, and safe words. Like any kink or fetish, it should be approached with respect and acceptance, without judgment or shame.

Sexual Asphyxiation

Sexual asphyxiation is a kink that involves the act of cutting off one's air supply for the purpose of enhancing sexual pleasure. It can be done solo or with a partner, and can involve various methods such as choking, strangulation, or the use of a breathing apparatus.

The origins of sexual asphyxiation can be traced back to ancient Rome, where it was believed that the loss of oxygen caused a heightened state of arousal. The practice became more popular in the BDSM community in the 20th century, and has since become a relatively common fetish.

Practitioners of this fetish enjoy the feeling of helplessness and intense pleasure that comes from the restriction of oxygen. It often involves a power dynamic, with one partner being dominant and the other submissive. However, it's crucial that those involved in this type of play establish clear communication and trust, use safe words, and avoid causing any physical harm or injury.

Similar kinks to sexual asphyxiation include breath control, choking, and even forms of autoerotic asphyxiation. However, it's important to note that these practices can be extremely dangerous and potentially life-threatening when done unsafely, without the proper precautions and preparation.

Ultimately, it's important to remember that all kinks and fetishes should be practiced safely and consensually. By being open-minded, respectful, and communicative with your partner, you can enjoy an intimate and fulfilling sexual experience. Don't hesitate to seek out resources or guidance if you're unsure about how to safely engage in this type of play.

Spanking

Spanking is a kink that involves striking someone's buttocks with an open hand or an object for the purpose of sexual pleasure or punishment. It can be practiced in different ways, ranging from light taps to intense blows that leave bruises on the skin. It is a form of BDSM play, and often involves a power dynamic in which one partner is dominant and the other submissive.

The origin of spanking can be traced back to ancient Greek and Roman times, where it was used as a form of discipline for slaves and servants. Over time, it became a common form of punishment in households and institutions, and later evolved into a popular kink within the BDSM community.

There are several practices associated with spanking, including role-play scenarios such as teacher/student, boss/employee, or parent/child. Spanking can also be combined with other BDSM activities such as bondage or sensory play to create a more intense sexual experience. It's important for those involved in spanking to establish clear boundaries and communication before engaging in play, especially when it comes to the intensity of the spanks and the use of objects.

Similar kinks to spanking include paddling, flogging, and caning, all of which involve striking the body with an object for sexual pleasure or punishment. However, spanking tends to be more common and less extreme than other forms of impact play.

It's important to note that not everyone is into spanking, and it's not a "normal" or necessary aspect of BDSM or sexual play. However, for those who are interested in it, spanking can be a fun and satisfying part of sexual exploration that can enhance intimacy and trust between partners.

In conclusion, spanking is a kink that involves striking someone's buttocks for sexual pleasure or punishment. It has origins in both historical discipline and BDSM culture and involves a power dynamic between partners. Safe and consensual communication is key to practicing spanking, and it's important to start slow and build up intensity while establishing boundaries and safe words.

Squirting

Squirting, also known as female ejaculation, is a sexual act that involves the release of fluid from the genitalia during orgasm. The fluid comes from the Skene's glands, a group of glands that are located near the G-spot in females. Squirting can be a source of pleasure and excitement for those involved, and it has become a common fetish in the porn industry and among certain sexual communities.

The origin of squirting has been debated by sexologists and researchers. Some believe that it has a biological purpose, while others suggest that it is purely for sexual pleasure. There is a significant lack of research on squirting, which has caused controversy over what exactly it is and whether it is a legitimate form of sexual expression.

Cheryl Bach

Squirting is typically achieved through G-spot stimulation, either through vaginal penetration or through other forms of sexual play such as fingering or using sex toys. It can also be achieved through clitoral stimulation, and some women are able to squirt without any external stimulation at all.

There are different practices associated with squirting, including techniques to help increase the likelihood of achieving squirting, such as prolonged stimulation of the G-spot or the use of specific sex toys. Some individuals may prefer to squirt directly onto their partner or onto themselves as a form of sexual expression or satisfaction.

Similar kinks to squirting include watersports or urophilia, which involves a fascination with urine and urination. However, squirting is generally considered to be a separate and distinct sexual practice that involves the release of fluid during orgasm.

Despite its popularity, squirting remains a controversial and somewhat taboo fetish. Some individuals may feel embarrassed or ashamed about their ability to squirt, while others may fetishize it to an unhealthy extent. It's important to approach this kink with compassion and respect for those involved, and to recognize that it is a legitimate form of sexual expression for some individuals.

Stockings and Hosiery Fetishism

Stockings and Hosiery Fetishism is a form of sexual fetishism that involves a strong sexual attraction to stockings, pantyhose, tights, and other types of hosiery worn on the legs and feet. This fetish can manifest itself in different ways, including through the act of wearing, touching, smelling, or admiring hosiery.

The origin of this fetishism is not entirely clear, but one theory is that it emerged during World War II when stockings were in short supply, causing them to become highly sought after and considered a luxury item. Today, fetishists may indulge in this fetish by collecting and wearing their own hosiery, or by seeking out partners who wear particular types of hosiery as part of sexual play.

Practices associated with hosiery fetishism typically involve the wearing, touching, or smelling of hosiery, either alone or in combination with other sexual activities. Some fetishists may derive sexual pleasure from simply admiring hosiery, while others may incorporate them into role-playing scenarios or BDSM activities. Hosiery worn on the feet may also be part of foot fetishism or shoe fetishism.

Similar kinks to stockings and hosiery fetishism include lingerie fetishism, which involves a sexual attraction to various types of underwear, particularly lingerie worn by women. While there can be overlap between the two fetishes, stockings and hosiery fetishism focuses specifically on the legs and feet. Additionally, foot fetishism or partialism specifically centers on the feet themselves rather than any object worn on them.

It's also important to remember that enjoying stockings and hosiery fetishism is a legitimate form of sexual expression and desire. However, it's important to ensure that any activities are consensual and respectful to all involved parties. Always consider your partner's boundaries and respect your own as well.

Suspension Bondage

Suspension bondage is a type of bondage that involves suspending a bound person in the air by rope or other restraints, often in complex or visually striking positions. This fetish is popular among BDSM practitioners, activists, and enthusiasts, who enjoy the challenge of manipulating the human body and pushing its physical limits to their boundaries.

The practice of suspension bondage has its roots in the shibari and kinbaku traditions of Japanese rope bondage, which have long been used for artistic expression and erotic play. Suspension bondage is now practiced by BDSM communities around the world, with enthusiasts creating intricate patterns of knots and ropes that both bind and support the suspended body.

Practices associated with this fetish include using complementary equipment like bondage bars, carabiners, and pulleys to create the right environment to suspend an individual safely, as well as following safety guidelines that include proper tying techniques and proper monitoring of the suspended person's breathing and pulse.

Due to the nature of suspension bondage, it is essential to ensure that safety is prioritized at all times. Suspension bondage can be dangerous if not done properly, such as when the rope or restraints used are too tight, or if the person being suspended has any pre-existing medical conditions that may be aggravated by being suspended in the air. It is important to research proper techniques and attend workshops led by experienced practitioners before attempting this fetish activity.

While suspension bondage may share similarities with other forms of bondage, such as rope bondage or metal bondage, it is a unique practice due to the complex nature of suspending a person in mid-air. Other related fetishes include self-suspension bondage, which involves an individual suspending themselves, and Shibari, which refers more specifically to the Japanese rope bondage tradition that is a foundational component of suspension bondage.

In conclusion, suspension bondage is a popular fetish within BDSM communities and involves suspending a person in mid-air with a system of ropes or restraints. It's important to remember that safety is paramount when practicing this fetish due to the potential for injury, and that proper research and education is essential. As with any fetish, communication and consent are essential, and partners should be comfortable with all aspects of the activity before proceeding.

Tentacle Fetishism

Tentacle fetishism is a sexual fetish that involves a strong attraction to images or depictions of tentacles. This fetish originated in Japan through various forms of media but has since spread to other parts of the world. Although this fetish objectifies tentacles, which are typically associated with sea creatures, it does not involve an attraction to the creatures themselves.

The origin of tentacle fetishism can be traced back to Japanese erotic art known as "shokushu goukan" or tentacle erotica, which depicted sea creatures or monsters engaging in non-consensual sexual acts with women. These depictions inspired the creation of anime and hentai featuring tentacles as well. However, in modern times, the representation of tentacles shifted from non-consensual acts to consensual and mutually pleasurable experiences.

Tentacle fetishism can be practiced in different ways. One common way is the consumption of animated media where tentacles or tentacled monsters play a significant role in sexualized scenarios. Another way is through literature, visual art, and photography, where tentacles are depicted in erotic ways. Some individuals enjoy incorporating sex toys such as tentacle shaped dildos or masturbators into their sexual experiences.

It's worth noting that tentacle fetishism shares intersections with other fetishes such as bondage, domination, and submission. The tying of tentacles around the body of one partner to subdue and control can be seen as an act of BDSM. It should be also mentioned that tentacle fetishism is not solely limited to heterosexual interests.

It's important to understand that while tentacle fetishism may seem odd to some people, it still falls under the umbrella of valid and consensual sexual desire, and individuals who engage in it should not be shamed or ostracized. Tentacle fetishism can also serve as a way for people to explore their desires in a safe and consensual manner free from judgment.

It's crucial that individuals engaging in tentacle fetishism understand how to explore this activity safely. If incorporating sex toys, it's essential to adhere to the manufacturer's guidelines. Additionally, it is vital to have clear communication with any partners involved to ensure that the practiced activities are consensual and comfortable for all parties.

To conclude, tentacle fetishism is a fetish that originated from Japan and involves an attraction to tentacles present in various media like literature, visual art, and animated media. The fetish has evolved over time and is no longer limited to non-consensual acts, but it's important to adhere to safety guidelines and communicate with all partners involved. While it may not be understood by everyone, tentacle fetishism is just another form of consensual sexual expression and should be respected as such.

It's worth noting that while there may be some similarities between tentacle fetishism and other fetish subcultures, each fetish has its unique characteristics, and individuals should educate themselves on the specifics of each one before engaging.

Whether or not one chooses to engage in tentacle fetishism, it's important to maintain open-mindedness and tolerance towards those who do. It's essential to understand that sexual desires and interests can be diverse and influenced by a variety of factors, and it is not up to us to shame or judge others' consensual choices.

Transvestism

Transvestism is a sexual fetish that involves wearing clothing that is typically associated with the opposite gender. This fetish is often linked to a desire to express oneself in a different way or feel a sense of empowerment by deviating from societal norms of gendered dress and appearance. However, it's important to note that not all individuals who cross-dress have a transvestism fetish, and vice versa.

The origin of transvestism can be traced back to different cultural practices throughout history, such as cross-dressing in theater performances or religious ceremonies. In more recent times, the subculture of drag and cross-dressing gained visibility through LGBTQ+ movements. Similarly, the practice of transvestism has evolved over time and has become more widely accepted as an expression of gender variance rather than a fetish subculture.

Transvestism can take different forms, including private dress-up sessions at home, public performances in drag shows, or even incorporating gender-bending clothing into everyday life. Some individuals may go to great lengths to create a convincing appearance of the opposite gender, while others may wear less elaborate attire. It's important to note that for some individuals, transvestism may not be a sexual act, but rather a form of self-expression.

It's worth noting that transvestism shares intersections with other fetishes and kinks such as sissification or feminization. These involve emasculation and submission, whereby individuals experience pleasure in being degraded and forced to conform to stereotypical gender norms. However, it's important to understand that not all transvestism involves emasculation or submission, and these individuals should not be lumped together or judged as one category.

In conclusion, transvestism is a form of sexual expression that involves wearing clothing typically associated with the opposite gender. It has a rich cultural history and can be seen as a way to express oneself or challenge societal norms of gendered dress and appearance. While it may share similarities with other fetishes and kinks, it's important to understand that not all individuals who cross-dress have a transvestism fetish, and vice versa.

Urolagnia

Urolagnia, also known as "watersports," is a sexual fetish that involves urine play. This can manifest in a variety of ways, including urinating on oneself or others for sexual pleasure, being urinated on, or drinking or ingesting urine. While this fetish is considered taboo by many people, it is still a valid form of consensual sexual expression for some individuals.

The origin of urolagnia is not entirely clear. Some speculate that it may have originated from societal taboos and the thrill of breaking them, while others believe it may have roots in the ancient Roman practice of urophilia. Regardless of its origin, individuals who engage in urolagnia often describe it as a physically and emotionally arousing experience.

Urolagnia practices can vary greatly depending on the individuals involved and their preferences. Some may engage in golden showers, where one partner urinates on the other, while others may incorporate urine play into BDSM scenes, such as using it as a form of degradation or humiliation. It's important to note that all forms of urolagnia should be practiced with clear communication, consent, and safety measures in place to prevent the spread of infection.

While urolagnia may be considered taboo by some, it shares intersections with other fetishes and kinks that involve bodily fluids, such as coprophilia (feces play) or emetophilia (vomit play). However, it's important to differentiate between each fetish and understand the unique risks and considerations involved with each one.

In conclusion, urolagnia is a sexual fetish that involves urine play. This taboo fetish has roots in ancient practices and is still a valid form of consensual sexual expression for some individuals. While it may share intersections with other fetishes involving bodily fluids, it's important to understand the unique risks and considerations involved with urolagnia. As with any sexual expression, it should be practiced with respect and safety measures in place.

Voyeurism

Voyeurism is a sexual fetish that involves obtaining sexual pleasure from watching others engage in sexual activities or being naked. This can manifest in a variety of ways, including peeking through windows, spying on people having sex, or even watching pornographic material. While this fetish is considered taboo by many people, it is still a valid form of consensual sexual expression for some individuals.

The origin of voyeurism is not entirely clear. Some speculate that it may have originated from societal taboos and the thrill of breaking them, while others believe it may have roots in the ancient practice of spectacles, where people would gather to watch public sexual performances. Regardless of its origin, individuals who engage in voyeurism often describe it as a physically and emotionally arousing experience.

Voyeurism practices can vary greatly depending on the individuals involved and their preferences. Some may engage in peeping or spying on others without their knowledge or consent, while others may engage in consensual voyeurism with willing participants. It's important to note that voyeurism without consent is illegal and can be harmful to the individuals being watched.

While voyeurism may be considered taboo by some, it shares intersections with other fetishes and kinks that involve watching or being watched. For example, exhibitionism involves getting sexual pleasure from exposing oneself to others, while scopophilia involves watching or gazing at others for sexual pleasure. However, it's important to differentiate between each fetish and understand the unique risks and considerations involved with each one.

Additionally, it's important to understand the legal implications of voyeurism. In some jurisdictions, voyeurism may be criminalized and can come with severe consequences. It's essential to be aware of local laws and regulations before engaging in voyeuristic activities.

In conclusion, voyeurism is a sexual fetish that involves obtaining sexual pleasure from watching others engage in sexual activities or being naked. While it may be considered taboo by some, it can be a valid form of consensual sexual expression for those involved.

Wet and Messy Fetishism

Wet and Messy fetishism, also known as sploshing or WAM, is a sexual fetish that involves getting sexual pleasure from being covered in, or covering someone else in, various non-harmful substances, such as food, mud, paint, slime, or water. This fetish can manifest in a variety of ways, from playful and lighthearted to more intense and extreme acts of degradation or humiliation.

The origin of wet and messy fetishism is not entirely clear. Some speculate that it may have originated from ancient practices of using food and other substances in sexual rituals, while others believe it may have roots in BDSM practices involving domination and submission. Regardless of its origin, individuals who engage in wet and messy play describe the sensation as unique, arousing, and often liberating.

The practices involved in wet and messy fetishism can vary greatly depending on the individuals involved and their preferences. Some may engage in light, playful activities like food fights or sploshing, while others may engage in more intense acts of degradation or humiliation. Partners may take turns covering each other in substances or use props like a pie or cake to enhance the experience.

Wet and messy fetishism shares intersections with other fetishes and kinks that involve sensory play or bodily fluids. For example, spitting and salirophilia both involve arousal from bodily fluids, while haptic sensory play involves the use of touch and sensation to provoke sexual pleasure. However, it's important to differentiate between each fetish and understand the unique risks and considerations involved with each one.

One important consideration when engaging in wet and messy play is hygiene. Individuals should ensure that the substances used are non-toxic and not harmful to skin or eyes. It is also important to clean up thoroughly after play and avoid food products that may cause infections. Communication and consent are also crucial to ensure that all participants are comfortable with the substances used and the intensity of the play.

Some practical tips for exploring wet and messy fetishism include starting slow and building up intensity gradually with a trusted and consenting partner, using non-toxic substances to avoid irritation or allergy, and being mindful of cleanliness and hygiene to avoid infections or health concerns. It's also important to have open communication about boundaries and desires to ensure a safe and enjoyable experience for all involved.

Cheryl Bach

Whipping

Whipping is a BDSM practice that involves the use of a whip or similar implement to inflict pain on the body of a consenting partner. It can be used as a form of punishment in a dominant/submissive dynamic, or as a form of sensory play, enhancing sexual arousal through pain and sensation.

The origin of whipping in BDSM is not entirely clear, but it has been present in human sexual history for centuries. Some believe it originated from ancient flagellation rituals, while others attribute it to the practices of slave masters during the slave trade. Regardless of its origin, individuals who engage in whipping describe the sensation as unique, invigorating, and even spiritual.

Practices involved in whipping can vary greatly depending on the individuals involved and their preferences. A dominant partner may use a whip or flogger to deliver strikes to areas of the submissive's body, such as the buttocks, back, or thighs. It's crucial to establish communication, consent, and safe words before engaging in any form of BDSM play. The intensity and frequency of strikes can be increased or decreased, depending on the desires of both partners. Whipping can also be combined with other BDSM activities such as bondage or sensory deprivation.

Whipping shares intersections with other BDSM practices that involve pain and submission, such as caning or spanking. However, it's important to differentiate between each practice and understand the unique risks and considerations involved with each one. For example, caning can cause more severe injuries than whipping, while spanking may not involve the use of an implement at all.

When exploring whipping, it's important to consider safety measures. The use of a safe word is crucial, as it allows the submissive partner to communicate when the experience is too intense or uncomfortable. It's also important to establish boundaries beforehand and to agree on a safe strike zone (areas of the body that are safe to strike) to avoid causing permanent damage or injury. The Dominant partner should also be aware of the force and the intensity of their strikes and take breaks as needed.

Some practical tips for safely exploring whipping include starting gradually, communicating regularly, using a safe word, and avoiding areas with major organs or nerves, such as the neck, spine, or genitals. It's also important to ensure that both partners are sober and not under the influence of drugs or alcohol.

In conclusion, whipping is a BDSM practice that involves the use of a whip or similar implement to inflict pain on a consenting partner. While it can be an intense and potentially dangerous activity, when practiced safely and consensually, it can enhance sexual pleasure.

Xenophilia (attraction to aliens or non-human entities)

Xenophilia is a sexual fetish that involves an attraction to non-human creatures or entities. It is sometimes referred to as monster fetishism, and may involve attraction to science fiction creatures such as aliens, werewolves, or mermaids. While it may seem like an obscure kink, it is actually quite common, and can be explored through various forms of media, such as video games, cartoons, and literature.

The origins of xenophilia in sexual fetishism are difficult to trace, given the diversity of media representations throughout history. People who are attracted to non-human entities may be drawn to elements of escapism, power dynamics, or unique, sensational experiences. The practice of using otherworldly or anthropomorphized characters in sexual fantasies is not novel, but with the advent of technology and the vast degree of access to different types of media, it has become more widely accepted and discussed.

Practices involved in xenophilia can range from solo fantasies to roleplaying with a partner. Some individuals may collect figurines or artwork depicting their ideal creature, while others may engage in sexual acts with toys or full-body costumes that resemble their preferred species. Consent and communication are critical when practicing any form of fantasy or fetishism, and it is important to understand that all parties involved are consenting adults and that no one is being objectified or exploited.

Xenophilia can be compared to other fetishes that involve attraction to seemingly non-human creatures, such as furry fetishism. However, it is essential to note that xenophilia is not inherently associated with the furry community and can exist independently.

When exploring xenophilia fantasies, it's important to approach them with an open and curious mind. Safe exploration can include discussing your fantasies with a trusted partner, and incorporating them into role-playing or dirty talk. As with any kink, there are risks to be aware of, such as the potential for cultural insensitivity or objectification of marginalized groups. Practicing sensitivity and respect for the beliefs and cultures associated with different creatures or entities is key.

Practical tips for safely exploring xenophilia fetishes include establishing clear boundaries and sticking to them, utilizing safe words, communicating consistently, and researching safe sex practices associated with costume play or toy use. It is also essential to acknowledge the difference between fantasy and reality and to understand that while these creatures may not exist in real life, consent, respect, and safety are always necessary when exploring these fantasies.

In conclusion, xenophilia is a sexual fetish that involves an attraction to non-human entities, such as aliens or mermaids. While it may seem strange to some people, it is a relatively common kink that can be explored safely with consenting partners. As with any fetish or kink, communication and consent are essential, and it's crucial to establish boundaries beforehand. While there are risks involved in exploring this fantasy, there are also many practical tips that can help keep you safe and ensure that you have a pleasurable experience. Overall, it is important to approach this or any other kink with an open mind, respect, and safety at the forefront of your exploration.

Chapter 4

The Psychology of Kinks and Fetishes

Kinks and fetishes are a complex and fascinating aspect of human sexuality that has been the subject of scientific and psychological study for decades. There are many theories as to why people have kinks and fetishes, including biological, psychological, and social factors.

Theories behind Kinks and Fetishes

Kinks and fetishes are believed to stem from a combination of biological, psychological, and social factors. One explanation is through the process of conditioning or association between a specific stimulus and erotic arousal. People may also develop fetishes as a way to cope with negative experiences.

Classical Conditioning: Classical conditioning theory suggests that people develop kinks and fetishes through repeated exposure and association with a particular stimulus. For instance, a person may develop a foot fetish through positive experiences with foot stimulation.

Operant Conditioning: Operant conditioning theory proposes that our behaviors are influenced by reinforcement and punishment in our environment. People may shape their behaviors to fit into social norms based on external forces.

Biological Factors: Biological factors such as hormones, genes, and brain chemistry can also influence an individual's sexual desires. For instance, hormones like testosterone and estrogen can play a role in fetishes and kinks.

Psychological Factors: Psychological traits like personality, attachment style, and history of trauma can also play a role in the development of kinks and fetishes. For instance, individuals with insecure attachment styles may seek out power dynamics in their sexual relationships as a way to feel more secure.

Social Factors: Social factors such as cultural norms, upbringing, and media exposure can also influence one's sexual desires. For example, societal stigma around certain sexual acts or desires can lead individuals to hide or suppress their fetishes.

Myths and Misconceptions

Despite increasing acceptance and understanding of kinks and fetishes, there are still many myths and misconceptions surrounding this aspect of human sexuality. Myths and stereotypes can perpetuate stigmatization, shame, and misunderstandings about kinks and fetishes, making it difficult for people to explore their desires and find acceptance. Common misconceptions include that kinks and fetishes are unnatural or abnormal, that they are linked to mental illness or trauma, or that people with kinks and fetishes are inherently dangerous.

Scientific Research on Kinks and Fetishes

Recent scientific research has explored the biology and psychology behind human sexual desires, including kinks and fetishes. Studies have suggested that different types of fetishes involve distinct patterns of brain activity, and that there may be genetic or hormonal factors influencing kink development. However, more research is needed in this area to fully understand the complex interplay between biology, psychology, and social factors in shaping sexual desires.

Individual Experiences

In addition to these broader factors, individual experiences and upbringing can also shape one's sexuality, including kinks and fetishes. Personal experiences, traumatic events, upbringing, and relationships with caregivers and partners can all play a role in shaping one's sexual desires. For example, sexual abuse in childhood may lead to certain fetishes or aversions later in life.

Overcoming Shame and Stigma

Despite the growing understanding of kinks and fetishes, it can still be difficult for individuals to explore their desires and find acceptance, particularly due to social stigma and shame. Overcoming this stigma requires individual acceptance, self-exploration, and non-judgmental communication with partners. It is important to create a safe and supportive space for exploration and to communicate boundaries and consent clearly.

In conclusion, our sexual desires, including kinks and fetishes, are influenced by a complex interplay between biological, psychological, and social factors. These desires are shaped by our personal experiences, upbringing, cultural norms, and external stimuli. Despite the stigma and myths surrounding kinks and fetishes, it is essential to create a safe and non-judgmental space for self-exploration, communication, and consent. Sexual exploration can be a positive and healthy aspect of human experience, enhancing intimacy, pleasure, and connection between individuals.

Chapter 5

Incorporating Kinks and Fetishes in Your Sex Life

Whether you have been exploring your kinks and fetishes for a while or are just beginning, incorporating them into your sex life can be both exciting and challenging. When done properly, it can enhance intimacy, passion, and pleasure in your sexual experiences. However, it requires self-awareness, open communication, and a willingness to explore new territory. In this chapter, we will provide practical tips on how to embrace your kinks and fetishes, communicate your desires with partners, and practice safe and consensual sex.

Embracing Your Kinks and Fetishes

The first step in incorporating your kinks and fetishes into your sex life is accepting yourself. It is essential to embrace your kinks and fetishes rather than feel ashamed or embarrassed about them. Self-acceptance will help you to communicate your desires more effectively, which is key to incorporating your kinks and fetishes into your sex life.

Once you have accepted yourself, it is important to educate yourself on your kinks and fetishes. This involves researching the activities, understanding the risks involved, and learning how to practice them safely. Joining fetish communities or attending workshops and events can also help you get a better understanding of your kinks and fetishes.

Cheryl Bach

Communicating Your Desires

Talking about your sexual desires takes courage and vulnerability, but it is essential for effective communication and consent.

Here are some tips for effectively communicating with your partner(s):

Start small: Begin by talking about your desires in a non-sexual setting, such as during a casual conversation. This can help to avoid any pressure or expectations.

Be specific: Use descriptive language when communicating your desires to your partner. The more specific you are, the more your partner can understand your needs and work towards fulfilling them.

Use "I" statements: When discussing your kinks and fetishes, use "I" statements to avoid making your partner feel defensive.

Active listening: Listen actively and non-judgmentally when your partner is sharing their desires as well. This helps to build trust and foster healthy communication.

Check for understanding: Confirm with your partner that you have understood their desires correctly and ask any clarifying questions.

Practicing Safe and Consensual Sex

Safety and consent are essential when it comes to incorporating kinks and fetishes into your sex life.

Here are some tips to ensure that you practice safe and consensual sexual activities:

Establish clear boundaries: Discuss and agree on boundaries before engaging in sexual activities. Ensure that both partners understand and respect each other's limits.

Cheryl Bach

Use safe words: Safe words are an essential tool for indicating when a partner needs to stop or reduce an activity. They allow partners to communicate effectively during sexual activities.

Do not pressure your partner: It is essential not to pressure your partner into any sexual activity, especially ones that they are not comfortable with.

Practice safer sex: This involves using contraception and protection against sexually transmitted infections (STIs).

Take care of aftercare: Aftercare involves taking care of oneself and one's partner after a kinky or fetish-related activity. This can include physical comfort such as providing water, cuddling, and emotional support.

It is important to note that consenting adults must agree to engage in kinks and fetishes, and all participants must have the necessary information, resources, and communication skills to make informed decisions.

Advice for Individuals New to Exploring their Kinks and Fetishes

For those who are new to exploring their kinks and fetishes, the process can feel overwhelming.

Here are some tips for beginning your exploration:

Start with self-exploration: Before discussing your desires with a partner, it is helpful to start by exploring your own body and what sensations give you pleasure.

Take things slowly: It is important to take things slowly and gradually when exploring your kinks and fetishes. This can help you identify what activities you enjoy and how far you are willing to go.

Be open-minded: As you begin to explore, be open to new experiences and activities that you might not have considered before.

Attend fetish events and workshops: Going to events and workshops can help you learn more about your kinks and fetishes and meet others who share similar interests. This can be a great way to learn from experienced individuals and build confidence in exploring your own desires.

Build trust with your partner: It is important to build trust and mutual respect with your partner before engaging in any kinky or fetish-related activities. This is crucial for establishing clear boundaries and ensuring that all parties feel safe and comfortable.

Remember to take breaks: Exploring kinks and fetishes can be an emotionally and physically intense experience.

Remember to take breaks and prioritize self-care in order to avoid burnout and fatigue.

In summary, incorporating kinks and fetishes into your sex life can be a rewarding and fulfilling experience. However, it requires self-awareness, open communication, and a commitment to safety and consent. By embracing your desires, communicating effectively with your partner(s), and practicing safe and consensual sex, you can enjoy healthy and fulfilling sexual experiences.

Chapter 6

Legal Issues and Taboos

Individuals who have unusual or unconventional sexual interests often feel a sense of shame, isolation, or fear of being judged. In addition to the psychological issues, there are also legal risks that should be taken into consideration when considering exploring one's sexual desires. This chapter will explore the legal issues surrounding kinks and fetishes, as well as examine the historical taboo on certain sexual practices, and the cultural variations in regards to sexual practices.

Legal Issues Surrounding Kinks and Fetishes

It is important for individuals who have kinks and fetishes to understand the legal risks associated with their interests.

Most countries have laws that regulate sex work, pornography, and prostitution. These laws often carry severe penalties for those involved in these activities, including fines and imprisonment.

Individuals may also face legal issues stemming from general criminal statutes, such as assault, battery, and sexual harassment. In cases where the partner involved in the kink or fetish activity is not a consenting adult, legal ramifications can arise. The use of BDSM equipment or toys may also be restricted and individuals may face criminal charges for possessing such items.

It is important for individuals to understand their local laws and regulations regarding sexual activity and to ensure that any activities they engage in are consensual and legal. Engaging in illicit or non-consensual activity can lead to severe legal consequences.

Cheryl Bach

Global Attitudes towards Kinks and Fetishes

Attitudes towards kinks and fetishes vary greatly across different cultures. In some parts of the world, sexuality is still considered a private matter and engaging in any unconventional sexual practices is considered taboo.

In other cultures, such as certain parts of Europe, Japan, and the United States, there is a greater tolerance and understanding of individuals with alternative sexual preferences. In these cultures, kinks and fetishes may be viewed as just another aspect of sexuality and are generally more accepted.

However, even in cultures that are generally more accepting of kinks and fetishes, there can still be legal and social stigmas attached to certain practices. It is important for individuals to research and understand the cultural norms and legal regulations in their area before engaging in any activities that are outside of mainstream sexual practices.

Historically Taboo Kinks and Fetishes

Throughout history, certain sexual practices have been considered taboo and even punishable by law. For example, homosexuality was once criminalized in many countries and considered a mental disorder until the 1970s.

Other kinks and fetishes such as BDSM, cross-dressing, and voyeurism have also faced criminalization and social stigmas throughout history. It is important to recognize and understand the historical context behind these stigmas and to work towards dismantling them through advocacy and education. As attitudes towards sexuality continue to evolve, it is important to reflect on past discrimination and prejudice and work towards building a more sex-positive world.

Cheryl Bach

Cultural Variations in Regards to Sexual Practices

Cultural differences can greatly impact attitudes towards sexuality and sexual practices. For example, many cultures have specific sexual practices that are considered normal or even revered.

In certain parts of India, for example, tantric sex is a respected tradition that involves deep spiritual connection and energy exchange. In Japan, bondage and restraint have long been a part of erotic art and literature. It is important to recognize and appreciate these cultural differences while also ensuring that any activities engaged in are safe, consensual, and legal.

In conclusion, understanding legal issues and taboos related to kinks and fetishes is crucial for individuals considering exploring their sexual desires. It is important to research and understand local laws and regulations, as well as cultural attitudes towards sexuality in order to ensure that any activities engaged in are consensual, safe, and legal.

Historically taboo kinks and fetishes have faced oppression and discrimination, and it is important to recognize and work towards dismantling these stigmas. Cultural variations in regards to sexual practices should be respected and appreciated while also ensuring that all parties involved are consenting adults.

By understanding legal risks, historical contexts, and cultural attitudes, individuals can better navigate the world of kinks and fetishes and safely enjoy their sexual desires.

Chapter 7

Healing and Therapy

It is not uncommon for an individual's sexual preferences to be influenced by their past experiences, specifically those that were traumatic or negative. These experiences can range from physical and emotional abuse to neglect or abandonment. In this chapter, we will explore how past traumatic experiences can impact one's sexual preferences, how individuals can seek healing and therapy to address their concerns, and the many forms of therapy that may be used to help individuals struggling with sexual issues.

How Past Traumatic Experiences Can Impact Sexual Preferences

Traumatic experiences can have a significant impact on an individual's sexuality and sexual preferences. For example, a person who experienced sexual abuse may develop a kink or fetish related to the type of abuse they experienced, such as BDSM or role-playing.

Additionally, a person who experienced emotional neglect or abandonment may seek out relationships or engage in specific sexual acts as a way to feel validated and loved. These experiences can also lead to sexual dysfunctions such as erectile dysfunction or difficulty achieving orgasm.

It is important to understand that these preferences and behaviors do not make an individual immoral, disgusting or wrong. Rather, they are a manifestation of how the individual has learned to cope with their past experiences. It is important to have a healthy and non-judgemental attitude towards these individuals and offer them the support they need.

How Individuals Can Seek Healing and Therapy to Address Their Concerns

Seeking therapy or counseling is an important step towards addressing past trauma and the related sexual issues. A qualified therapist or counselor can help individuals work through their feelings, develop coping mechanisms and strategies, and ultimately achieve a healthier and happier life and sex life.

To seek therapy, an individual should research and find a licensed and experienced therapist who specializes in working with sexual trauma and related issues. The therapy sessions can be conducted either individually or in a group setting.

It is important to choose a therapist who is non-judgmental and empathetic, and who creates a safe and supportive environment for the patient. In some cases, the therapist may also work with the individual's partner(s) to address relationship issues associated with the past trauma.

The Many Forms of Therapy That May Be Used to Help Individuals Struggling with Sexual Issues

Many different forms of therapy can be used to help individuals struggling with sexual issues related to past trauma.

Some popular examples include:

Cognitive-behavioral therapy (CBT): This form of therapy focuses on helping individuals change their thought patterns and behaviors to develop healthier coping mechanisms. It can be beneficial for individuals struggling with sexual dysfunctions or experiencing anxiety related to sexual experiences.

Cheryl Bach

Eye movement desensitization and reprocessing (EMDR): EMDR is a form of psychotherapy that has shown to be effective in treating trauma-related issues. It involves guided eye movements which can help process traumatic memories and reduce their impact on the patient's present life and functioning.

Somatic therapy: This approach emphasizes the connection between the body and the mind, working to release stored emotional responses and physical tension associated with past trauma. This is usually done through techniques like massage, yoga, or other forms of bodywork.

Talk therapy: Many individuals find relief from talking about their experiences and emotions. That process may look like group therapy, art therapy, psychological education/explanation, reflective writing etc.

Hypnotherapy: This form of therapy involves the use of guided relaxation, visualization, and suggestion to help bring up the traumatizing experience, unearth buried memories, and help the individual work through them in a safe and structured manner.

It is important to note that there is no one-size-fits-all approach to therapy, and what works for one individual may not necessarily work for another. It is important to find a therapist and therapy-type that suits an individual's specific needs and preferences.

In conclusion, past traumatic experiences can negatively impact an individual's sexuality and sexual preferences. However, it is important to understand that seeking help and going through therapy can lead to long-lasting healing and personal growth.

There are various forms of therapy that individuals can choose from to address and work through past trauma. Whatever approach it might be, it is crucial to understand that the work can be difficult and challenging, yet it can lead to positive change, a better understanding of self, and better sexual relationships.

In the end, whether you are dealing with past trauma or supporting someone who is, it is important to approach the situation with compassion and empathy. Trauma can have a lasting impact on an individual's life, but therapeutic interventions can help to reduce symptoms and increase quality of life. With time and patience, it is possible to work through past trauma and find a fulfilling and satisfying sex life.

Chapter 8

Kinks and Fetishes Online Resource

Thanks to the internet, there are countless online resources where individuals can explore and share information about their kinks and fetishes. In this chapter, we will discuss websites, online forums, social media groups, and other platforms that cater to the kink community. We will also examine how individuals can navigate fetish and kink dating sites.

Websites, Online Forums, and Social Media Groups Related to Kinks and Fetishes

The internet is full of communities, websites, and online forums where people can discuss and engage with their sexual preferences. Some popular websites include FetLife,

Alt.com, and Collarspace, all of which provide a platform for exploring and discussing different kinks and fetishes.

FetLife, in particular, is a social media platform designed specifically for the kink community. Users can create profiles, join groups, post pictures, and share information about their kinks and fetishes. It is a great resource for connecting with others who share similar interests and for finding events in your area.

Alt.com is another popular website that caters to the BDSM community. It offers a variety of features, including chat rooms, webcams, and user-generated content.

Collarspace is a website that focuses on connection through BDSM. It offers a chat feature, a list of local events, blogs, and articles related to power exchange and sex.

Social media platforms like Reddit and Tumblr also have active communities for kink enthusiasts. These sites offer an opportunity for individuals to engage with like-minded individuals, ask questions, and find resources related to their kinks and fetishes.

Navigating Fetish and Kink Dating Sites

Fetish and kink dating sites can be a bit overwhelming to navigate, particularly for those who are new to the kink community. Here are a few tips on how to make the most of these sites:

Choose a site that caters to your specific interests: There are a variety of fetish and kink dating sites available, so it's important to choose a site that caters to your specific interests. Some sites focus solely on BDSM, while others allow users to search for partners based on specific kinks or fetishes.

Be honest about your interests: Honesty is always the best policy, particularly when it comes to kink and fetish dating. Be upfront about your interests and preferences, and don't be afraid to state your boundaries.

Take your time: Finding the right partner can take time, so don't rush into anything. Take the time to explore the site, chat with different users and get to know them before meeting in person.

Use discretion: While it's important to be honest about your preferences, it's also important to use discretion when sharing personal information. Avoid sharing your full name or address until you feel comfortable with the other person.

Watch out for scams: Unfortunately, there are scammers and predators on every dating site, including kink and fetish dating sites. Be cautious of anyone who seems too good to be true, and never send money to someone you haven't met in person.

Communicate clearly: Communication is key in any relationship, but it's especially important in the kink community. Be clear about your boundaries and expectations, and make sure your partner is on the same page.

Chapter 9

Kinks and Fetishes for Couples

Kinks and fetishes are a normal part of human sexuality and can be an exciting way to explore one's sexual boundaries. But what happens when two people in a relationship have different kinks and fetishes? The key to developing a healthy appreciation for each other's kinks lies in open and honest communication.

In this chapter, we will explore how couples can develop a healthy appreciation for each other's kinks and fetishes, practical tips on how to incorporate different kinks into sex with one's partner and advice on how to formulate boundaries and safe words as a couple.

Developing a Healthy Appreciation for Each Other's Kinks

Couples who have been together for a while may have discovered that they have different kinks and fetishes. It is important to note that every individual has their preferences, and it is acceptable. The key to developing a healthy appreciation of each other's kinks is in open and honest communication.

When you communicate with your partner about your kinks and fantasies, ensure that you approach the conversation in a non-judgmental manner. Be respectful of your partner's preferences, even if they don't align with your own. The goal should not be to change your partner but to understand and embrace each other's sexual preferences.

It is also important for couples to explore each other's kinks gradually and in a safe and consensual way. Starting small and building up can help prevent any discomfort or unsafe situations from arising. It is essential to establish boundaries and safe words to ensure that both partners feel comfortable and secure during any sexual activities.

Incorporating Different Kinks into Sex with One's Partner

Once both partners have a better understanding of each other's kinks and fetishes, it's time to start incorporating them into your sexual activities. This can be done gradually, starting with something simple and slowly working towards more complex scenarios or fetishes.

It is important to start with activities that both partners are comfortable with. For example, if a partner is interested in BDSM, starting with light bondage or sensory play can be a great way to explore this kink together. When trying out new activities, it is important to communicate wants and needs clearly to prevent any misunderstandings and keep both partners safe.

Experimenting with different kinks and fetishes can also be a great way to spice up a couples' sex life. Consider using sex toys, role-playing, or fantasy scenarios to help bring different kinks into the bedroom. Always remember to take things slow and be respectful of each other's limits and boundaries.

Formulating Boundaries and Safe Words as a Couple

Once both partners have agreed to explore different kinks and fetishes, setting boundaries and safe words is an essential step towards ensuring a safe and enjoyable experience.

Boundaries should be set to help establish what is and isn't okay in the context of the sexual activity. Couples should discuss what acts they are comfortable with, and what is off-limits. Examples of boundaries include limiting certain types of physical contact or only engaging in certain activities under specific conditions. It is important not to push your partner to do something they are uncomfortable with.

Safe words are also essential in any sexual activity that involves kinks or fetishes. A safe word serves as a signal for the partner to stop what they're doing immediately. When picking a safe word, avoid words that might be confused with moans or pleasurable noises. A simple and easy-to-remember phrase that is not typically used in sexual scenarios makes an excellent safe word.

Chapter 10

The Future of Kinks and Fetishes

In this chapter, we will discuss society's evolving awareness and acceptance of kinks and fetishes, how changes in technology and media are impacting how individuals explore and discuss their kinks, and what the future may hold for kinks and fetishes.

Society's Awareness and Acceptance of Kinks and Fetishes

In the past, kinks and fetishes were often shrouded in secrecy or considered taboo. However, with changing societal attitudes towards sexuality and more open discussions about different kinks and fetishes, people today are more accepting and less likely to judge those who engage in these activities.

Many factors have contributed to this paradigm shift, including the growing acceptance of sexual diversity and LGBTQ+ rights. Additionally, the increased education and awareness of consent and safe, responsible sexual practices has led to a greater understanding of kinks and fetishes that emphasizes mutual, consensual exploration. As a result, individuals are becoming more open about their kinks and fetishes, leading to a broader acceptance in society.

Impact of Technology and Media on Exploration of Kinks and Fetishes

Advancements in technology and media have also impacted how individuals explore and discuss their kinks and fetishes. The internet has made it easier for individuals to access information and connect with others who share similar interests. Social media platforms and online forums have allowed for open discussions about kinks and fetishes, as well as providing resources for individuals who may feel isolated or unsure about their desires.

Moreover, advancements in sex toy technology are allowing individuals to experiment with different kinks and fetishes both alone and with partners in a safe and controlled environment. In addition, the rise of virtual reality and other immersive technologies is creating new opportunities for exploring and simulating different kinks and fetishes.

However, it's important to note that this increased accessibility to kinks and fetishes through technology and media can also create potential risks and dangers. For example, some individuals may feel pressured into exploring kinks and fetishes they are uncomfortable with due to peer pressure or unrealistic expectations portrayed online. It is essential that individuals always remember to prioritize their own safety, wellness, and consent when exploring these activities.

The Future of Kinks and Fetishes

As society becomes more open and accepting towards different sexual practices, it's likely that kinks and fetishes will continue to evolve and become more accepted. With technological advancements, individuals may have even more opportunities to explore their desires in new and creative ways.

However, it is also important to recognize that everyone's journey with kinks and fetishes is unique, and there will always be people who do not understand or accept these practices. It is essential to continue conversations about consent, safety, and respect when exploring kinks and fetishes.

In the future, we may see further advancements in sex toy technology and virtual reality, creating even more opportunities for individuals to explore kinks and fetishes with partners or alone. It is also possible that we may see more government regulations or restrictions on certain kinks and fetishes.

Remember that as long as you prioritize safety, wellness, and consent, there are endless possibilities for exploration and pleasure. Keep an open mind, and never be afraid to communicate your desires with your partner(s).

Chapter 11

Conclusion

We have reached the last chapter of the Kinks and Fetishes Handbook. In this final chapter, we will recap the benefits of embracing one's kinks and fetishes, provide a message of support to those exploring their sexual preferences, encourage open and honest communication with partners about kinks and fetishes, and offer some final thoughts on the importance of accepting and loving oneself.

Recapping the Benefits of Embracing One's Kinks and Fetishes

Embracing one's kinks and fetishes can have numerous benefits, including increased self-esteem, improved communication with partners, and more fulfilling sexual experiences. When individuals allow themselves to explore their desires without judgement, they can fully embrace their sexuality and discover new ways to experience pleasure and connection.

Moreover, exploring kinks and fetishes can also expand one's understanding of themselves and others, leading to more empathy, respect, and openness in all aspects of life.

A Message of Support for Those Exploring Their Sexual Preferences

For those who are exploring their kinks and fetishes, it is important to remember that there is no shame in embracing one's desires. Everyone has different needs and interests, and it is essential to prioritize one's safety, wellness, and consent above all else.

Cheryl Bach

Whether you are just starting to explore your kinks and fetishes or are a seasoned practitioner, know that you are not alone. There are communities and resources available for individuals at every stage of the journey.

Encouraging Open and Honest Communication with Partners about Kinks and Fetishes

Open and honest communication is essential when it comes to exploring kinks and fetishes with partners. It is essential to establish clear boundaries, discuss preferences and limits, and continually check in with partners to ensure everyone is comfortable and consenting.

It can be difficult to initiate these conversations, but it is essential to remember that communication is key to a healthy, fulfilling sex life. By having these discussions, individuals may discover new ways to connect with their partners and deepen their intimacy.

It is also important to remember that individuals have the right to say no and set boundaries at any time, even during sexual activity. It is never okay for a partner to pressure someone into doing something they are not comfortable with.

Final Thoughts on the Importance of Accepting and Loving Oneself

Embracing and exploring one's kinks and fetishes is an essential part of accepting and loving oneself. By accepting and embracing all aspects of oneself, including desires that may be stigmatized by society, individuals can live more authentic, fulfilling lives.

It is essential to prioritize self-care and self-love when diving into the world of kinks and fetishes. This includes setting personal boundaries, taking breaks as needed, and engaging in activities that promote wellness such as meditation, exercise, or spending time outdoors.

Moreover, individuals should never feel ashamed or judged for their kinks and fetishes. Everyone has different desires and needs, and it is important to respect and celebrate this diversity.

In conclusion, the world of kinks and fetishes is vast and diverse. By exploring one's desires with an open mind and prioritizing safety, wellness, and consent, individuals can discover new ways to experience sexual pleasure and intimacy. It is essential to communicate openly with partners about kinks and fetishes, and never feel ashamed or judged for embracing one's sexuality. Embracing and loving oneself is the key to living a fulfilling, authentic life in all aspects. So embrace your kinks and fetishes, communicate with honesty and respect, prioritize self-care and self-love, and enjoy the journey of discovering all that your sexuality has to offer. Thank you for reading the Kinks and Fetishes Handbook, and we wish you all the best in your sexual exploration and growth!